HOMO...

A Patient's Guide

An introduction to homoeopathy, a system of medicine
founded by Samuel Hahnemann nearly 200 years ago and
now rapidly regaining its popularity. Dr Clover describes
homoeopathic prescribing today and discusses the thinking
behind the therapy.

HOMOEOPATHY

A Patient's Guide

by

Dr Anne M. Clover
Consultant in Homoeopathic Medicine

THORSONS PUBLISHERS INC.
New York

Thorsons Publishers Inc.
377 Park Avenue South
New York, New York   10016

First U.S. Edition 1984

LIBRARY OF CONGRESS CATALOGING IN PUBLICATION
DATA

Clover, Anne.
   Homoeopathy, a patient's guide.

   Bibliography: p.
   Includes index.
   1. Homeopathy—Popular works.   I. Title.
[DNLM: 1. Homeopathy—popular works. WB 930 C647h]
RX76.C66   1984   615.5'32   84–8549
ISBN 0–7225–0892–1 (pbk.)

Printed and bound in Great Britain

Thorsons Publishers Inc. are distributed to the trade by
Inner Traditions International Ltd., New York

Contents

Acknowledgements

I would like to express my thanks to Dr Michael Jenkins and Dr Trevor Cook for the helpful comments they made when checking initial drafts of this guide, also to Mrs Beryl Best and Miss Rachel Pellett for their efficient and careful assistance in typing its pages.

Finally, may I record my deep gratitude to Mr Eugene Halliday for his guidance and encouragement to research the deeper as well as perhaps better-known implications of homoeopathy.

Introduction

Today, when the name homoeopathy is mentioned in conversation it is often met with interest, questions and comments. It is a notable change from times as recent as twenty or even ten years ago when reference to homoeopathy was more likely to evoke blank stares of utter non-comprehension.

Many illustrations could be given of this growth of interest in the subject. Examples are the repeated references to it in the media, the proliferation of societies of people keen to support the understanding and availability of homoeopathy, the increasing numbers of doctors seeking post-graduate training in the speciality, and above all, the surge of requests from patients seeking homoeopathic treatment. All these factors illustrate the widespread acceleration of interest in the subject and demand for its availability.

Two factors appear to have contributed to this. The first is a positive interest in the subject itself and what it has to offer. This part of the twentieth century has witnessed a general increase in therapeutic methods and life styles sometimes termed 'alternative' or 'natural'. It reflects a positive swing towards such therapies and related concerns such as diet, that are regarded as natural and easier to assimilate than some of the more technical or synthetic contemporary products. It

appears to be part of a polarization of attitudes. The last few
decades have witnessed, on the one hand, a remarkable
growth in scientific and technical achievements and, on the
other, a surge of interest in simpler life styles, diets and
therapeutic methods. Extreme illustrations of this are
computer-controlled houses contrasting attempts to live the
'good life'; supermarkets proffering vast ranges of convenience
foods sited next door to wholefood stores and stalls; and high
technology-medicine developing alongside expanding depart-
ments of acupuncture and homoeopathy. They are all illustrations of the twentieth century polarization.

Whilst one aspect of this surge of interest in homoeopathy is
a positive interest in the subject for its own sake, another is,
unfortunately, disillusionment with the side-effects of modern
technological medicine. The advances and advantages of
modern chemo-therapy, surgery and related disciplines are
obvious, but so too are its side-effects. This is unfortunate but
it has to be acknowledged. Not infrequently patients are heard
to say 'I would rather have the disease than the side-effects of
the treatment'. Such disillusionment is another factor leading
many people to enquire further about other therapies, sometimes called 'alternative' medicine.

The term 'alternative' may have misleading implications if
it is taken to imply that the therapies associated with it are
seen as an 'either/or' in relation to conventional or orthodox
practices. Such an interpretation would be regarded by most
homoeopathic doctors today as erroneous. A better term being
used increasingly today is 'complementary therapy'. It is
better in that it implies that homoeopathy can be used as an
adjunct to many other non-toxic therapies. There are often
occasions when homoeopathy can be the main therapy
required to assist healing, but in many other situations it
affords a useful additional string to the therapeutic bow. Now-
a-days it is increasingly acknowledged that most diseases are
the result of diverse causal factors. It follows from this that
various lines of therapy may well be appropriate to help with

healing. Hence the value of a term like 'complementary therapy' which reminds us of this fact.

So, as we pursue this brief study of homoeopathy, we will consider both the subject itself and the way in which it can be applied in co-operation with other appropriate lines of therapy.

Chapter 1

Homoeopathy – What's in a Name?

A patient newly referred to a homoeopathic outpatient clinic recently walked in to see her doctor, sat down and announced that she wanted this form of treatment because it was 'natural'. Further discussion showed that she thought its medicines all came from herbs and that these were prescribed in small doses. Such ideas are widely held. Discussions about homoeopathy frequently illustrate the prevalence of these two ideas about the origin and dosage of homoeopathic medicines. The strength of such popular interpretations is often shown by the vigour with which they are expressed. But this does not mean they are entirely correct.

It is true to say that most homoeopathic medicines come from naturally occurring, rather than synthetic, products. Most come from plants such as aconite or monkshood. Many others come from minerals – gold is an example – and a smaller group from animal products, such as snake venoms. Such sources are often described as 'naturally occurring'. But there is also another small group of medicines derived from manufactured compounds. An example is an extract of gun-powder used to treat some types of eczema. The sources are many and varied and although the majority are natural products this cannot be said of all of them.

The other widely held idea concerns the size of the dose of such medicines. Many people think that homoeopathy means treatment with small doses. At a recent medical meeting a doctor who thought his colleague's prescription for a patient was too small described it as 'homoeopathic'. It is a common mis-use of the term homoeopathy.It is a mis-use on two counts: firstly, because the word homoeopathy does not mean small doses (its precise meaning will be discussed shortly) and, secondly, because the medicines prescribed in homoeopathy are not merely smaller-than-usual amounts of non-homoeopathic prescriptions. They are from different sources, selected on different principles and often prescribed in doses that are not merely small, but miniscule. More of this later.

What then does the name homoeopathy actually mean?
One of the easiest ways to begin to discuss the meaning of the name homoeopathy is to take it back to its Greek roots. It incorporates two Greek words, *homoios* and *pathos*. These are root forms that occur in many terms, but when placed together aptly summarize a method of prescribing. *Homoios* implies like or similar. We see it used again in such words as 'homogenous', meaning a similar kind of form so that a homogenous mixture has a smooth blended texture; and in homosexual, implying an attraction between people of the same sex. *Pathos* is also a commonly applied term. It means suffering and occurs in such words as pathetic or even in its anglicized form as pathos.

If, therefore, we put these two roots together we have a single term which implies 'like suffering' and neatly summarizes the basic idea on which homoeopathic medicine is founded.

At first this may appear a strange way to summarize a method that can be used for treating illness. But together the two words imply the practice of using an agent, that can cause symptoms in healthy people, to treat a similar condition when it is prescribed in a disease. It is like the old idea of having 'a hair of the dog that bit you'. To people familiar with homoeopathy this idea will be well known, but for some it may be a new thought and need more discussion.

Treating Likes With Likes

The idea fundamental to homoeopathic prescribing is that the agent used to treat symptoms occurring in the course of a disease can at other times produce similar affects if someone not suffering from the disease process takes a sufficient dose of the medicine concerned. It is often summarized by the saying 'let likes be treated by likes'. Or, expressing the same words in the Latin form often used by Samuel Hahnemann, a German doctor who pioneered the development of contemporary homoeopathic medicine, '*similia similibus curentur*'.

This saying is frequently quoted. It is a short way of advocating the use of an agent capable of producing symptoms to treat a *similar* change when it is part of a disease. The disease, and the agent that can treat it, both produce a *similar* effect. It is this use of similarly acting agents that is neatly summarized in those two Greek roots that comprise the name 'homoeopathy'. *Homoios* and *pathos* imply the similarity between the suffering in a disease and the effect of an agent that can mimic its symptoms.

The idea of treating 'likes by likes' is not limited to homoeopathic medical practice. When homoeopathy is discussed at meetings introducing the subject the comment is often made that this is also the basis of vaccination. Many of us have experienced this, despite vocal protests, in our first few months of life. We probably resisted with all our infantile muscle, but even so a minute dose given to us of modified agents that can produce diseases such as diptheria or tetanus have effectively increased our resistance to such infections. This type of therapy has, of course, differences from the use of homoeopathic remedies to treat already present disease. Preventive treatment, a prophylaxis, as it is technically known, is an application of the *similia* idea before the symptoms have occurred. Even so, it is a use of the organism associated with the cause of a particular illness to prevent its development in a person. The principle involved is closely related to the idea governing the use of a homoeopathic medicine to treat already existing disease.

It is not only in the treatment or prevention of infectious diseases that we find examples of treating likes with likes. We can find them in ordinary every-day events. An illustration is the practice of warming a burned hand to ease the pain of a burn or scald. It is a trick often advised by cooks. Such a simple act to reduce the pain of a burn again illustrates the idea that finds particular emphasis in homoeopathic medicine.

We will shortly look at the implications of using *similars*, as they are sometimes known, in more detail. But before we come to this let us take two examples of common diseases and plants able to mimic their symptons or treat them. This will then lead us more easily into a further discussion of the idea basic to homoeopathic practice. Our two examples will be the common cold and onion; and acute feverish illness and Deadly Nightshade. The onion is a vegetable commonly used and well known for its effect on the nose and eyes. Many of us find when peeling an onion that the membranes lining the eyes and nose frequently produce tears or a streaming watery discharge. In highly sensitive people the eyes can become red and sore with this reaction and the tears be profuse. Such a reaction will be familiar, probably to most of us. We will also easily recognize its similarity to the symptons of the common cold. Which brings us straight away to an illustration of the *similia* principle fundamental to homoeopathy. An onion can produce cold-like symptoms; when an extract of a red onion is prepared and dispensed homoeopathically it can often effectively treat such changes. The botanical name for the red onion is *Allium cepa*. Using this botanical name, which makes international recognition easier, an extract of the onion prepared according to the method used in homeopathic pharmacy is widely dispensed for certain types of common cold infection. The method of prepartion and presentation of the onion extract are subjects of later chapters, at the moment the idea of it is introduced simply to illustrate an application of the *similia* principle.

Another example of this principle, or using likes for likes, occurs with *Atropa belladonna*, popularly called Deadly Nightshade. This plant with its attractive bright red berries, is often found presenting a splash of colour in the countryside. Consequently children need to be warned not to be deceived by these attractive-looking fruits into thinking that they are good to eat. Unfortunately, however, an unwary or disobedient child at times succumbs to the lure of these berries and eats them. The results can be severe; these berries are highly poisonous and are capable of producing widespread, as well as serious, effects. Many books, as well as parental warnings, remind us that swallowing a few of these berries can quickly lead to severe dryness of the mouth, increased heat, thirst, excitability, flushed appearance and restlessness. Such symptoms readily compare with those produced by someone with an acute infectious illness such as measles. Children show this particularly clearly, often presenting early signs of producing a feverish illness by complaining of thirst, feeling hot and looking flushed. As is often said, the 'redness' is a particular feature of this condition. An infected area such as a tonsil may well look flushed or bright red, so too may the face of the child coping with it. In homoeopathic practice a prescription of *Belladonna* may be used here. It has often been reported to ease the effects of such feverish illnesses and to reduce the need for antibiotics.

There are, of course, reports of more severe degrees of poisoning from Deadly Nightshade swallowed accidentally. Unfortunately it can proceed to difficulty with swallowing or speaking, severe tightness of the throat, vomiting, delerium and even coma or death. Advanced stages of infectious diseases are rarely seen to-day in the West, but many books still remind us that such symptoms used frequently to occur with severe infectious illness. In earlier decades homoeopathic *Belladonna* was described as effective even in severe infectious disease producing the more florrid array of symptoms. A particular example was scarlet fever. There were many reports of homoeopathic *Belladonna* greatly easing the symptoms of this unpleasant disease. In a report published in 1801 entitled *Cure and Prevention of Scarlet Fever* Samuel Hahnemann outlines the preparation and use of an extract of *Belladonna* for this disease. He says:

> Three children in a family had succumbed to a very bad attack of scarlet fever; the eldest daughter, who had up to that time been taking *Belladonna* internally for some other external disease of the finger joints, was the only one who to my surprise refused to sicken with the fever, in spite of the fact that she was always the first to catch any other disease that chanced to be prevalent. After that I did not hesitate to give this providential remedy in very small doses to the remaining children of this numerous family as a preventive; but as the remarkable effect of this remedy does not last for more than three full days, I repeated the dose every seventy-two hours and they all remained well and were not attacked in the slightest degree throughout the whole epidemic although amongst the most poisonous odours from brothers and sisters who were still suffering from the fever . . . I concluded that a remedy which can speedily cure the beginning of an illness must be its best preventive.

It is interesting briefly to pause in our discussion of homoeopathy and look at the name *Belladonna*. The name comes from Latin roots meaning 'beautiful woman' and is said to refer to an ancient custom of putting some juice from the plant into the eyes to produce dilated and attractive pupils. At times aristocratic Egyptian women pursued this to such a degree that they impaired their sight. Homatropine, an extract of *Belladonna,* is still often used today in medical practice deliberately to produce temporary and safe dilation of the pupils to assist examination of eyes. This too can be another indication of how *Belladonna* can be used homoeopathically. When, for instance, a child has a raised temperature in an illness for which *Belladonna* may be suitable, one of the additional pointers to this is dilated pupils. Again, it is like for like. The illness which includes dilated pupils and other features similar to effects of *Belladonna,* may at times be suitable for treatment by an extract of a plant able to produce them.

These are just a few examples of the *similia* principle. There are, of course, thousands of them. In a later chapter on 'provings' we will discuss how the principle has been investigated deliberately by patients and doctors who have taken many substances from plant, mineral or animal sources in order to investigate or 'prove' their effects in human beings. Once these effects are carefully observed they can be correlated with symptoms occurring in disease, and extracts from them used where appropriate in therapy. They are all applications of using 'likes for likes', the idea fundamental to homoeopathy and implicit in its name.

The Origins of Homoeopathy

Having looked at this term 'homoeopathy' and considered a few illustrations of its application, people often ask – when and where did it start? The answer to this question lies far back in history. Early references to the idea can be found in ancient Greek medicine. The writings of Hippocrates for example contain references to agents that can cause disease being capable of helping to overcome it. Hippocrates was writing in approximately 400BC. He is sometimes called the 'Father of Medicine' since one of his major activities was to establish a school for physicians. Perhaps this was one of the first schools to teach homoeopathy. Another source of early references to the idea of homoeopathy is the writings of Paracelsus. These come from the early sixteenth century and are therefore recent when compared to the works of

Hippocrates. Paracelsus suggested that since diseases can be caused by agents that in other circumstances could treat them, the disease and the medicine to treat it should have the same name.

But even though such early references were made to the idea of using agents that cause illness to treat it, only through the work of Samuel Hahnemann in the late eighteenth and early nineteenth centuries has this practice become established in a form applicable in the medical scene today.

The present-day practice of homoeopathy continues to apply the *similia* principle usually with very dilute extracts of the medicine it indicates for a particular disease. Many examples could be given by patients and prescribers of its effectiveness in a wide range of conditions. Parents often find it helpful in treating children or themselves for minor injuries or infection. Reports are often given of how healing of cuts and bruises or common infections, such as influenza and colds, have been helped by homoeopathic treatment. Other problems for which homoeopathic medicines can be very helpful include longer-lasting diseases, technically described as chronic. Common examples are arthritis, eczema and migraine. Remedies that may be advised for such diseases are a direct application of the *similia* principle. Substances that could induce joint pains, irritant skin eruptions and headaches similar to those occuring in such diseases are used to treat them. Eczma is an illustration particularly easy to understand. Many people know all too clearly that frequent handling of petrol or oil can produce a dermatitis in sensitive individuals. The eruption of irritant patches with cracks in the skin is often similar to that occurring in patients with eczema from other causes. A homoeopathic medicine often used successfully in the treatment of such irritant eczema is petroleum. In the specially prepared dilutions used in homoeopathy this medicine had helped many people with this unpleasant condition. It is a direct application of the *similia* principle that is as valid today as it was when first researched and described by Dr Samuel Hahnemann.

It is sometimes said that 1796 saw 'the birth of homoeopathy'. In that year Samuel Hahnemann first wrote for public reading about the *similia* principle, or as he called it, the 'similia' law. At the same time he introduced the term 'homoeopathy' to describe the practice founded on it.

In an Essay on *A New Principle for Ascertaining the Curative Powers of Drugs and some Examinations of the Previous Principles* Hahnemann writes:

> One should imitate nature, which at times, heals a chronic illness by another additional one. One should apply in the disease to be healed, particularly if chronic, that remedy which is able to simulate another artificially-produced disease, as similar as possible, and the former will be healed – *similia similibus* – likes with likes.

This was written when Hahnemann was forty-one years old. He did much more writing after this, expressing his continuing search for a greater understanding of such ideas and their implications. Throughout his writings there is a gradual clarification of the rationale for treating likes with likes and how this can be applied in practice. The *Organon*, one of Hahnemann's major works, is particularly concerned with the ideas on which homoeopathic medicine is founded. The fact that there are six editions of this book, first published in 1810 and with the final edition written shortly before his death in 1843, and published posthumously, illustrates Hahnemann's own application to the continual search for a greater understanding and better application of the ideas of *similia* therapy.

Although Hahnemann revises his understanding of the *similia* principle recurrently as he writes, the fundamental idea remains constant. He continuously restates that the agent that can cause disease can be used to treat it. This basic tenet holds firm but at the same time his consideration of it becomes increasingly profound. Like so many other statements, the *similia* idea can be taken at face value and applied, for instance, in the treatment of certain types of common cold infection by a homoeopathic extract of onion. That is the superficial application. But to the deeply enquiring mind of Hahnemann such an interpretation was worthy of extension. As well as noting the effect, he asked its cause. In many writings subsequent to the statement of the *similia* principle Hahnemann repeatedly questioned the precise nature of diseases and the methods of therapy used in their treatment.

Recurrently he examines the subject in relation to knowledge of disease, knowledge of the powers contained in medicine and knowledge of how to apply the medicines 'judiciously and effectively'. He constantly reminds us to ask first what can we learn about the detailed as well as superficial factors in causes of disease, what potentially healing powers are 'hidden' in medicines and how can these two insights be brought together for appropriate treatment.

Today such questions are still valid. Although the understanding of disease has increased since the day of Hahnemann we are still needing to ask such fundamental questions concerning all aspects of medicine.

How Does Homoeopathy Work?

What then can we say today about homoeopathic medicine and how it applies the idea of treating 'likes with likes'. To many people homoeopathy is a useful method of treatment. They find it effective and safe and that appears to be enough for them. But many others want to look further and question how it achieves its therapeutic effects, or to put it more simply, they say – 'how does it work?' It is a commonly seen polarization of attitudes. Some homoeopathic prescribers and patients say – 'we know from practice that it works, but precisely how, we cannot say' – and they appear ready to leave it there. For these people a continuing practice is based on the past experience of effectiveness. Such a policy is sometimes described as 'empirical', that is, experience-based. Other prescribers and patients, however, will try to discuss ideas of how these medicines achieve their effect. This is not easy as the extracts used are often of such high dilution levels that molecules of the original substance cannot be demonstrated in them. Hence much more subtle procedures will be required for assessment of the forces involved than the ordinary gross large molecule measurements usually available in laboratories today.

To begin to question how homoeopathy works and to attempt to formulate an understanding of its principles is in keeping with Hahnemann's approach. In all his writings he insisted that homoeopathy was a 'rational', that is, reasonable, system of medicine. He even called the first edition of the *Organon*, '*An Organon of the Rational Art of Healing*'. In this and in subsequent books he recurrently contrasted the limits to practice based on data collected from particular experiences of illness and their treatment, with the expanded application of practice founded on ideas that are deduced first and then applied to the sick-bed scene. His assertion was that sick-bed scences were usually fraught with emotion and biased by the particular state of the patients, the relatives and the people offering treatment. In contrast to this he suggested that careful reason, deducing ideas before application at a sick-bed, afford less biased principles to select and apply. Hahnemann put it strongly, contrasting 'prejudice' based on limited experience, against pure reason derived from careful deduction. Putting it simply, he said first form an idea, then put it into practice.

For Hahnemann, the ideas were clarified, applied in practice, further clarified, re-applied, and so on. His six editions of the *Organon*, as well as revisions of other works, show his personal commitment to this ideal. Today we could liken it to working out a new plan even for a familiar journey rather than merely repeating an old well-tried route. Obviously a plan of action may need re-assement if problems or boredom are encountered. The previous plan affords a basis for continuing clarification. This principle is still as valid now as it was for Hahnemann nearly two hundred years ago.

What, therefore, can be said in an attempt to begin to understand how homoeopathy works? This question will be the subject of a whole chapter later in this guide. But as it is also relevant here some ideas related to it will be introduced ready for subsequent expansion. The theories expressed by Hahnemann again afford a helpful starting point for such discussion. He suggestd that an appropriate *similia* remedy presented another stimulus similar to that causing a disease. But, and this is very important to his deductions, it was in a form to which the body could respond more effectively and so provoked a more appropriate reaction against itself. This contrary action (Hahnemann called it a 'counter-revolution') then overcame the effect of the medicine, plus at the same time, the disease process similar to it. In other words, he suggests that the stimulus from a medicine is deliberately intended to mimic the disease to be treated. The medicine is a disturbance-creating factor carefully selected to provoke the body to oppose it. When the effect of the medicine and disease similar to it are both overcome, healthy function is restored.

The example of treating some types of common cold infection by a homoeopathic preparation of *Allium cepa* will again illustrate the principle. It is as if the cold infection provokes a disturbance to which the body does not immediately offer an adequate opposition. The *Allium cepa* prescribed then provokes a stronger response to itself which overcomes the medicinal effect. As this response is similar to and stronger than that of the cold, it also corrects the prior-disease state.

This was Hahnemann's theory. Today we can augment and expand it by using simple basic ideas from some of the remarkable disclosures of modern science.

Today it is known that all so-called material objects, including our own bodies, are actually fields of energy behaving as if they are solid. The atoms that comprise apparently gross objects, science reminds us, are whirling zones of energy. With this idea in our minds it is much easier to begin to think of the human body, whether healthy or diseased, as made up of many cells, or relatively small energy patterns, linked together in the larger overall complex. Such an idea can sound too simple to some people, too revolutionary to others. Even if at first it sounds simple its implications are vast. If it sounds revolutionary we may still examine it further.

Many of us who today are trying to understand homoeopathy were trained in early years, for instance at school, to regard material bodies as fundamentally different from immaterial forms, such as thoughts and feelings, that might or might not influence the part that 'really' counts or matters, the physical organism. The puns are deliberate. Such ideas were imprinted in our memories to such a degree that we still believe, if we are not careful, that the gross material aspect of the body is the part that really counts.

One result of this can be an idea that disease only exists if it can be demonstrated under a microscope as abnormal cells, or in a laboratory as abnormal levels of chemistry. Fortunately that attitude is changing. Increasingly it is accepted that in many diseases there are processes that still need correction even though laboratory data cannot be produced to describe in coarse terms what is happening. We know now that disease can be a disturbance of personal function and health although there may be no gross pathology or an apparent physical explantion for it. Psychiatric and psychosomatic illnesses are particularly clear examples of this principle. There may not be biochemistry or gross pathology to prove 'depression', but many patients, their relatives and doctors still see clear evidence of how this disease impairs personal function and health.

Such changes in a personal energy field frequently occur and can result in obvious symptoms affecting thought processes, emotional reactions or physical performance. They are clear examples of energy flow changes that are associated with disease even though gross cellular changes cannot always be defined to account for them. The process may be fairly easily recognised in relation to psychiatry but it also reminds us that even when an illness includes an apparantly defined change in cells, like inflammation of tonsils in tonsillitis, here also the changes are due to zones of energy behaving in this way. It is a change in the complex of body energy patterns and not merely particular gross cells reacting in this way.

Another reminder that the body cannot be adequately accounted for in terms merely of anatomical forms described from inspection under a microscope or chemicals measured in laboratory tests, is the frequently presented evidence of the ways in which ideas and feelings can determine physical behaviour. Modern psychology describes this interaction by referring to a 'three-part man'. It says that all of us are all the time influenced by the way we think, by our feelings and by physical habits. This triad is described technically as the interaction of the intellect, affect and physical drive. Illustrations of its validity are constantly occurring. Too little or too much food can affect a person's emotional and physical state; excitement or depression can influence his thinking and physical performance; thinking about something he enjoys can positively lift his emotions and help him in a task he is performing. Examples of this are occurring in every moment. If someone finds a letter to say he has won a large sum of money, he is highly likely to experience a faster pulse and produce a whirl of ideas on what to do with his prize. Conversely, a demand from the IRS can produce a very different effect. They are simple examples, but readily illustrate the way in which all aspects of the human body work together in every moment.

In rather more precise terms it is saying that our bodies are fields of energy where the processes of thought, feeling and physical pursuit are like currents converging in a single river. The functions of organs such as kidneys and lungs cannot be separated out, neither can the influence of such factors as emotion and thought. Remembering that even apparently gross organs are zones of energy appearing to be solid in form makes it much easier to think of the body as a complex of force fields co-operating in a particular system.

Such an understanding of the body composition opens the way for more dynamic assessments of diseases that are otherwise commonly associated with an over-emphasis on gross organs or chemical agents. It implies that any disease is a disturbance of the body energies and is a change that to some degree influences the whole system, even though at times it may appear to focus on a particular part. If we see the body as a continuous system of energy, disturbance in one aspect will to some degree be felt throughout its entirety. There may be relative stress on a selected organ, but there cannot be isolation. In considering methods of treating disease this implies the advantages of those that can help us with re-adjustment of psychological as well as physical aspects of the process. Obviously if someone has acute appendicitis they are likely to need surgery. But even this can be presented in a way which allows for adjustment of associated psychological reac-tions.

If we now apply these ideas to our considerations of homoeopathy we can see that they strongly support its appropriate use. It is arguable that the fine stimulus of a homoeopathic medicine can suitably provoke a reaction by psychological as well as physical energies of the patient. As noted earlier in this chapter, Hahnemann suggested that such a reaction against the stimulus of the medicine could then at the same time overcome the similar disturbance of all aspects of the original disease pattern. Hahnemann recurrently referred to treating the whole picture presented. The ideas now discussed are adding to his views a twentieth-century assessment and relating it to treating intellectual and emotional as well as physical aspects of the process.

Hahnemann wrote his books long before 'three-part man'

was described. But in many ways he anticipated the ideas to be made clearer later in the development of medicine and philosophy. Hahnemann said recurrently that in assessing a disease process the need is to look at the whole picture presented and try to understand the thought processes as well as the physical changes. He also emphasized the need to treat causes of disease as well as their physical effects. Perhaps he was working towards ideas now being made clearer through modern science. As he said recurrently, and others have since echoed in other ways, examining the gross state of organs is not enough thoroughly to explain or treat disease.

Hahnemann anticipated the discovery to be made after his death concerning the fact that all the organs that can be seen are the end products of subtle energy fields such as volition, intellect and emotion, that all the time determine their processes. Hence, it may be argued, the need for a therapy that can help with adjustment of the subtle as well as the gross energies that operate all the time in our bodies.

Homoeopathy, it may be said, is one such therapy. Later chapters will include discussion of how the idea of using a *similia* related to gross effects as well as causes of disease can be applied in practice.

This chapter began with the question – what is implicit in the name 'homoeopathy'? A brief answer says it is a summary of the *similia* principle fundamental to all the theory and practice of this form of medicine. It literally spells out, admittedly in Greek roots, the ideas on which this method of treatment is founded.

Another way of clarifying an understanding of the *similia* principle is through a brief resumé of Hahnemann's initial discovery and subsequent pursuit of it. This will be the subject of the next chapter.

Chapter 2

Hahnemann's Discovery of Homoeopathy

In the introduction to this guide it was noted that today's growth of interest in homoeopathy can be attributed both to an interest in the subject for its own sake and a degree of disillusion with some aspects of modern medicine. The same could be said about Hahnemann's discovery of the practice. He protested strongly about what he saw as deficiencies in the medicine of his day and at the same time sought alternatives. Various biographies written about him, as well as his own writings in case reports, books and papers reveal the intensity with which he sought for a new, effective and safe method of treating disease conditions.

In the late eighteenth century practices such as purging and blood letting were widely used in the treatment of disease. It was assumed that releasing fluid from the body in blood or by forced evacuation of the bowels would somehow assist the expulsion of the disease. Hahnemann protested strongly and clearly against such practices. He said that far from overcoming a disease, it weakened the body's reaction against it and therefore made the situation worse. His criticisms of such practices occur throughout his writings. They are usually lengthy and blunt. For instance, in the introduction to the *Organon*, Hahnemann writes:

In recent times the old school practitioners have quite surpassed themselves in their cruelty towards their sick fellow-creatures, and in the unsuitableness of their operations, as every unprejudiced observer must admit, and as even physicians of their own school have been forced, by the pricks of their conscience, to confess before the world.

With statements like this being published in his name perhaps it is hardly surprising that from the beginning of his work, Hahnemann and homoeopathy met with strong opposition from many medical colleagues.

Such negative factors were not the only driving force for Hahnemann. Whilst he spoke out against practices that he saw damaging to health he was also searching for better alternatives. His biographies tell how in 1791 at age thirty-six years Hahnemann came across a report that provoked him into a personal experiment as part of that continuing search. The experiment was to prove an important link in the chain of events that in due course led Hahnemann to deduce the *similia* principle.

The particular piece of research that appears to have led Hahnemann into homoeopathy arose out of translation work. His biographers describe how in the early 1790s Hahnemann was translating Cullen's *Treatise on Materia Medica* when he came across reports on the effects of Peruvian bark. They referred particularly to the effect of Peruvian bark in reducing the recurrent temperature peaks experienced by patients suffering from 'ague', the illness probably known today as malaria. Hahnemann disputed Cullen's account of how Peruvian bark was said to act and in order further to test it out gave himself doses of china, an extract of the bark, for a few days. He then observed that china produced in himself symptoms similar to those that occurred in people who had malaria. From his medical training he knew that in his day Peruvian bark was widely used to treat malaria. Putting these two observations together he deduced that Peruvian bark, or china, could treat malaria because of its capacity to cause similar symptoms in a healthy person. This was the year 1791. Five years later, after further explorations of the idea that diseases can be treated by agents capable of producing similar symptoms, Hahnemann published his views in an essay and coined the term 'homoeopathy'. The ideas were revolutionary. From the start they provoked both interest and opposition.

The sequence of events leading up to, through and beyond the china experiment is a remarkable example of scientific tenacity. Hahnemann had read reports of an observed effect, tested it out on himself, deduced a principle and then applied it to other situations. After his own initial experiments he recruited other interested people to assist him. Together they began to experiment with an increasing number of substances. Hahnemann compiled the reports and they became the early contents of his *Materia Medica*. It was the dawn of the modern practice of homoeopathy. In subsequent years more people became interested and joined the team of researchers into his new practice. The *similia* principle had been observed, reported and to an increasing degree was being applied.

The Provings

In the following years an increasing number of substances were taken by defined healthy volunteers to clarify their effects. Such experiments became known as 'provings'. They were intended to 'prove' the effects of medicines when taken by human beings. Following on from this, and as a direct application of the principle fundamental to homoeopathy, the reported effects could then be matched with symptoms of particular diseases. The agent that could mimic a disease could also be used to treat it. The terms coined by Hahnemann to describe this process are still widely used today. The experiments were termed 'provings'; the volunteers who had taken the medicines, 'provers'. The standards required by Hahnemann from his provers were rigorous. Some of his writings include his directions to provers. Amongst these are the directives to avoid alcohol, over-exertions of body or mind and even to keep free of 'all disturbing passions'.

Placebo Effect

When provings are discussed today a problem often raised concerns the modern understanding developing about 'placebo' effects. These had not been observed in Hahnemann's time so it would be unreasonable to criticize him for omitting reference to them. But today it is a well-known process and needs comment.

Placebo effect refers to the change that can be produced more by expectation than from a biological effect of medicines. Or, putting it technically, it is a response to medicine from psychological rather than physiological aspects of the human body. There are many examples of this response. Young children show it clearly when they believe any injury can be cured by 'a special plaster'.

The anticipation of an effect of a medicine may include, for instance, a state of fear, or eagerness or even an unconscious desire to leave this world. Today it is known from scientific experiment that emotions produce specific chemicals in the human body and modify its physical structure. In other words, the way we feel changes our physical state. This observation makes it much easier to accept and understand that the emotional states of people taking medicines can help or hinder their biological effects. The anticipation can either reinforce or retard the physical effects of medicine and influence the highly individual responses sometimes seen to widely used preparations.

It means, for instance, that the child who believes that a 'special plaster' will quickly help his cuts and bruises to heal actually speeds up his recovery because the idea and feeling he has about it changes his body chemistry in a helpful manner. Unfortunately the effect can also apply in an opposite manner. When, for instance, someone believes that no matter what treatment they have their illness will persist, that sort of idea and negative emotion also produces its own chemical effect and slows down the healing process.

In provings today, one way of allowing for such reactions, and yet still continuing with the tests to obtain the information needed for prescribing, is to work with very large groups of provers. If a high percentage of a large group of provers produce similar effects from a named medicine, they are likely to be associated with the power of the medicine itself to produce such changes in a human being rather than with an individual's reactions to the stimulus.

Toxicology

In a later chapter we will consider in more detail the way in which toxicology, or studies of the effects of poisonings, can assist homoeopathic prescribing. At the moment let us simply observe that it again applies the *similia* principle. Accidental, or deliberate, poisoning can serve as a type of proving. Two examples, often quoted in homoeopathic books from Hahnemann and his successors, are arsenic and mercury. Both of these substances were widely available for use in the time of Hahnemann. Arsenic was used as an ingredient in dyes or as a preservative, as well as perhaps for more sinister intent. Mercury was widely used in the treatment of syphilis.

Although there were examples of the judicious use of these agents there were also many reports of poisonings from accidental or even deliberate overdoses. It is not only doctors and chemists who have described the effects of arsenic. This has also been done, often with vivid detail, by crime writers. As a result it is widely known that the effects include progressive anaemia, restlessness, severe tiredness, stomach pain, diarrhoea and vomiting. Applied homoeopathically, this means that arsenic, in a suitably prepared form and dose, has been used to treat certain types of gastro-enteritis, stomach ulceration and anxiety.

Mercury has also been well-known for its poisonous effects, particularly from overdoses in attempts to treat syphilis many years ago. It has also been reported that symptoms similar to those now attributed to mercurial poisoning were found in men mining the ore from which mercury is abstracted. These symptoms, as well as those of syphilis and their exacerbation by mercury overdose, were known in Hahnemann's time. The toxic effects reported then, and still observable today, resemble the results of arsenic poisoning in that they again include severe diarrhoea and vomiting. However, with mercury there is also a particularly strong effect on the skin, bowel lining, salivation, tongue and gums. Having recognized these effects, Hahnemann used extracts of mercury, prepared according to homoeopathic principles, in the treatment of conditions such as diarrhoea, rectal bleeding from ulceration, mouth ulceration and skin disorders. These are just two examples of known toxic effects that can be recorded and applied homoeopathically. There are many others. Such reports when collected by Hahnemann and the colleagues who joined him added to the data from provings and gradually built up the homoeopathic prescribing manuals. That is, the *Materia Medica*.

Ultramolecular Dilution

As many of the substances used by early homoeopaths were highly toxic in their crude state, it is not surprising to find reports that even when, as Hahnemann directed, the dose was the 'smallest possible', at times there were aggravations of symptoms before an improvement. As the agent being taken could produce a similar effect to the already present disease, it is hardly surprising that at times there was an initial worsening of the condition. Such deteriorations were brief and said by Hahnemann to be evidence of a close fit between the disease and the prescribed medicine. Therefore, he said they were to be welcomed as the herald of a prompt improvement to follow. But even allowing for the insight that aggravation anticipates improvement of disease, most doctors and patients still prefer to avoid such upsets. Hahnemann also preferred to avoid them.

His writings indicate that attempts to reduce the aggravation led him to use progressively smaller doses of the selected medicine. He found that this still preserved the benefit but reduced or even averted the initial aggravation. Which brings us back to the small doses for which homoeopathy is to some famous, to others, infamous.

It has already been noted in the first chapter that the widely used doses of homoeopathic medicine are frequently not merely small, but miniscule. To put it technically, they are ultramolecular. A fuller discussion of this very important aspect of homoeopathic medicine is the subject of the next chapter. At this stage we are seeing how, for Hahnemann, it was a progressive development of his conviction that the dose needed was to be sufficiently small enough to avoid either toxic effects or aggravations of the prior disease, yet sufficiently powerful to provoke healing. He recurrently referred to the Hippocratic principle 'Above all do no harm'. Hahnemann's opening statement in the *Organon*, the book which refers particularly to the concepts on which homoeopathy is founded, reminded physicians that their first duty is to aim for a cure as rapidly, effectively and safely as possible. At the start of the *Organon* he says:

> The physicians's high and only mission is to restore the sick to health, to cure, as it is termed. The highest ideal of cure is rapid, gentle and permanent restoration of the health, or removal and annihilation of the disease in its whole extent, in the shortest, most reliable, and most harmless way, on easily comprehensible principles.

With this ideal goading his research, his prescribing used progressively smaller and smaller doses. Yet still they worked. Hence he went on with it, the extractions became finer, and eventually the use was established of the ultramolecular dilutions widely prescribed today. The dilution factors, and other processes in the preparation, involved not mere half or quarter doses. They were reductions on a series of 1 in 10 or 1 in 100 parts. It was a major development not merely for homoeopathic prescribing, but arguably, because of its implications, for all medical practice.

The discovery that such ultramolecular dilutions could assist healing of disease was startling. Today its challenge to medical thought and practice is as great as in the time of Hahnemann. It is hardly surprising that Hahnemann's work commonly provoked other medical colleagues to show towards homoeopathy more opposition than positive interest. Both then and now homoeopathy has been dismissed by some people unable or unwilling to allow that such dilutions could be therapeutically useful. It is unfortunate that throughout the development of medicine there have been people ready to dismiss and oppose new developments because they themselves cannot understand how they work, or because they strongly contradict ideas previously held.

Even such an important medical practice as the attempt to avoid infection, asepsis as it is technically known, was initially opposed. Stalwarts of old ideas at first strongly resisted the advice of colleagues about thoroughly cleaning their hands before moving from one patient with obvious infection to another. Anaesthesia is another example of a technique now universally welcomed that at first met with strong opposition from some of the patients and medical men of that era. Frequently what may be a wise caution about practices new to a particular decade has turned into prejudiced opposition. If such resistance was not itself adequately opposed it would stifle progress.

Another example of how such resistance to new ideas and ways can be a hindrance occurred when an elderly lady whose home had been newly wired for electric rather than gas lighting, refused to turn on the switch. She insisted that she was not having anything to do with that 'new-fangled electricity'. She said she could not see it or smell it, did not understand it and therefore would not use it. Unless someone else flicked the switch on for her, she sat in the dark. It took many months to persuade her to reconsider.

Fortunately the resistance shown to the new ideas being expressed by Hahnemann did not deter him. He persevered and the use of minute dilutions of therapeutic agents selected and prepared in the way he pioneered has remained a fundamental feature of homoeopathy and a challenge to orthodox medicine.

In the next chapter we will take a closer look at how such homoeopathic medicines are prepared and presented.

Chapter 3

Potentization

Earlier chapters have contained references to the minute doses of medicine commonly used in homoeopathic practice. The intention now is to take a closer look at how these miniscule doses are prepared and presented. As noted earlier, it is this aspect of homoeopathic medicine that is particularly well known. Although the *similia* principle implicit in the name is the basis of homoeopathy, (Greek, *homoios* – similar; *pathos* – suffering), it is generally better known for its use of infinitesimally small doses of medicine. Hence the occasional use of the term homoeopathic in colloquial speech to refer to weak tea, coffee, etc. This aspect of homoeopathic medicine appears to fire both the imagination and the critism of many people and is therefore generally better known than the principle actually signified by the name.

This raises a question. Why is it that these minute doses attract such attention? Frequently they arouse either argument or even anger. A discussion of their use has at times provoked angry responses from people resistant to ideas that appear to oppose their own prescribing methods. The amounts of medicine commonly used in conventional medicine are massive in comparison to the homoeopathic doses, and conventionally trained people often find it difficult to accept that these minute prescriptions can possibly have any effect. Such doubts are common products of attitudes established in student years. For many other people the reaction has been interest, an acknowledgement that these minute doses appear to help towards recovery from disease, and a questioning of how they produce their effect.

It is arguable that the two vectors, positive and negative, that provoke or prevent interest in homoeopathy again operate in responses to a discussion of homoeopathic 'potencies', that is, the minute extracts of its medicines commonly employed. The positive factor is often related to an understanding that disease can be determined by subtle energies, such as psychological factors, or by the minute amounts of irritant to which some people show allergic reactions, as well as by relatively gross cellular damage, infection and trauma. Those who accept that psychological factors, minute doses of an allergen (i.e. something that triggers an allergic reaction) and other very fine stimuli can provoke disease, often seem more inclined to consider that similar fine stimuli in homoeopathic medicines can initiate the healing process. The negative factor contributing to an interest in homoeopathic potencies is, unfortunately, the common experience of side-effects from conventional drugs. At times, whilst the benefits from such medicines are obvious, so too are the side-effects. There are of course many other factors such as the high cost of convential drugs that can also stimulate such an interest.

How then are these medicines produced?

There are more than 2,500 homoeopathic medicines coming from a wide range of sources. Briefly summarized these include plants, minerals, animal products, diseased tissue or secretions, chemical compounds and extracts of conventional drugs. It is a very long list and still growing as new sources of remedies are researched. It is worth noting that there are over half a million plant species on the earth, yet only about five per cent have been examined for their healing properties.

Botanical Sources of Medicines

The plants are the largest group, representing the source of more than sixty per cent of all homoeopathic medicines. They include examples from many countries. For instance, the arnica extracts widely used in the treatment of bruising are derived from *Arnica montana*, or Leopard's Bane, a plant that grows in abundance on the lower slopes of the Swiss Alps. Another example is the buttercup which gives a homoeopathic medicine known as *Ranunculus bulbosus*, the botanical name of the plant, and used for instance in irritant skin eruptions such as shingles.

The medicines obtained from plants are usually known by the botanical name of the source. In our first chapter we referred to *Allium cepa* obtained from the red onion, and *Atropa belladonna*, from Deadly Nightshade. These are commonly occurring plants and the remedies they yield have wide use in homoeopathy. Although many of the plants used have obvious physical effects, such as the poisoning from Deadly Nightshade, or effects of onion on eyes and noses, some of them appear to be relatively inactive. *Lycopodium*, Clubmoss, is an example of this. Most physicians in Hahnemann's time regarded it as inactive. However, Hahnemann himself showed that after repeated serial dilutions and sucussions, i.e. rhythmic shakings with impact, it yielded a medicine useful in conditions as various as certain types of anxiety state, gastric disorder or kidney problems.

Other botanical sources of homoeopathic medicines are trees and bushes. Homoeopathic medicines are prepared from their barks, roots, berries, seeds, flowers or leaves. For instance, ripe hawthorn berries give *Crataegus*, used in some heart conditions; the rhododendron gives an extract widely used in arthritis. *Cinchona*, from the bark of a tree sometimes known as the quina (hence the name quinine for one of its products) was used by Samuel Hahnemann in his first recorded experiment with the idea of homoeopathy when he tested it on himself. Plants, shrubs and trees are the largest group in the sources of homoeopathic medicines.

Mineral Sources of Medicines

Although less numerous than botanical sources, several minerals are used to obtain widely prescribed homoeopathic medicines. Examples include well-known compounds such as calcium phosphate and common salt or mineral substances such as gold, silver, platinum and sulphur. The method by which medicinal extracts of these or other minerals are obtained will be described shortly. For the moment the examples are given merely to illustrate the wide range of sources of homoeopathic medicines.

Animal Sources of Medicines

Another group of remedies comes from animal products. A wide range of creatures from land and water, and sundry products from them can be used to produce homoeopathic medicines. A few examples may again illustrate the diversity. They include cow's milk, the shell of the oyster, the blue dye ejected from the ink-bag of a cuttle fish when it is disturbed, venoms or stings from wasps, bees and tarantula spiders, cat fur and horse and dog hair.

Nosodes

The use of diseased tissues to produce homoeopathic medicines is often compared to the preparation of vaccines. In homoeopathic practice they are known technically as 'nosodes'. One of the first to be prepared was *Tuberculinum*, an extract of pus obtained from a tubercular abcess. It is a slightly different application of the *similia* idea discussed in the first chapter. Briefly described it is the use of an extract from a disease product, such as pus, to treat another condition in which the symptoms are closely similar to those of the illness producing the pus. One example is the use of *Tuberculinum* to treat some kinds of recurrent throat and chest problems. Children with such problems have often shown a decreased frequency of infection and reduced need for antibiotics after treatment with homoeopathic *Tuberculinum*.

Allergens

A further source of homoeopathic medicines relates to another development of Hahnemann's application of the *similia* principle. This involves the use of agents that commonly cause allergic reactions in susceptible individuals. Such agents are known technically as *allergens*. Probably better-known is the term for the reactions they provoke, namely *allergies*. Common examples are grass pollens provoking hay fever or house dust causing asthma. In homoeopathic medicine minute extractions of such agents, or of other defined *allergens* have often appeared to increase an individual's tolerance of such irritants. It means for instance that some forms of hay fever improve after treatment by a homoeopathic extract of grass pollen.

Extracts of Modern Drugs

Another development of Hahnemann's pioneer work is the use of extracts of modern drugs to treat some of the side-effects commonly associated with such medicines, or for similar symptoms occurring in the course of another disorder. An example may help. Let us consider aspirin. Although many people are grateful for its help in relieving problems like the pain of rheumatoid arthritis, it is well-known that in some people one of its side-effects can include ringing in the ears and dizziness. These symptoms can occur in many conditions and an extract of salicylic acid, the technical name for aspirin, is one of the homoeopathic medicines that may be used to treat them. Another common side-effect from a modern drug is a skin rash produced in an appropriately sensitive patient who takes penicillin. A homoeopathic extract of penicillin has at times been found very useful in reducing such a reaction. Again it is a clear example of using likes for likes, or an agent that can cause symptoms, to treat them.

These are just a few examples of the sources from which homoeopathic medicines can be obtained. The list is very long. Many of the agents are highly poisonous in their crude state, others apparently inactive. But all of them, prepared according to the clinical method developed by Hahnemann, can be presented in a form that is non-toxic yet therapeutically active. The method, as noted earlier, was referred to by Hahnemann as 'potentization'. That is, it is a means of presenting the power or potency of the agent in a safe but effective manner to assist healing.

The Aim of Potentization

The methods by which potencies are prepared today from the initial solutions or extractions of the source materials are essentially similar to those advised by Hahnemann. The techniques have of course been updated and, in some instances, modern aids are used in producing the extractions from the source materials. The medicines are produced in accordance with the methods described in the *Homoeopathic Pharmacopoeia* published in Britain and the U.S.A. Some details of the methods vary with different manufacturers. Some of them still have major parts of the process, such as rhythmic shaking between dilutions, done by hand. Others have introduced mechanical aids to simulate this part of the process. As the purpose of this book is to introduce in an easy manner the subject of homoeopathy, a detailed review of manufacturing methods is not within its scope. In considering 'potentization' the aim is therefore to focus on the principles governing it, rather than to try to describe details of today's production methods.

As Hahnemann recurrently stated, the aim in potentization is to present the essential form of the medicine in a manner that can be easily utilized by a patient towards assisting healing of a disease. The aim in the production of homoeopathic medicines is to reveal the natural subtlety and essence of the source material which in turn match the subtlety and essence of the person receiving them. The six editions of the *Organon* in which Hahnemann expressed many of his ideas about how homoeopathic medicines work show that he was gradually clarifying an understanding that first there is an essential form of, for instance, a plant or mineral. This, he says, is a hidden 'dynamic radical'. It appears that he is suggesting that every natural form has a dynamic essence to which forces are added in time to give its ordinary gross appearance.

We could perhaps liken it to a person who wears a distinctive dress by which she becomes known, or to the genetic code of an embryo that determines the uptake of food and other solar energy in a certain manner so that one child appears tall, another short, and so on. Hahnemann's theory is that the essential determinant, or 'dynamic radical', is the most active part of the substance since it governs the gross presentation seen in the material world. In his later writings he referred to this structure as a 'spirit-like essence'. This, he suggests, is 'unveiled', as the translator expresses his German, in the process of potentization. He coined the term 'potency', or more accurately, its German equivalent, to convey the idea of the powerful radical central to the structure of, for instance, a belladonna plant or onion bulb. The process of 'potentization' is then said to unveil or reveal this dynamic form and present it in a way that can help stimulate healing in a diseased body.

How Potentization is Achieved

The process by which he advised carrying out this unveiling includes serial dilutions of the original solution interspersed with rhythmic, vigorous shaking with impact on a hard surface. Hahnemann achieved this by a rhythmic movement of his arm and striking the vial on a leatherbound book. But nowadays the process is often simulated in a specially designed machine.

Let us take first the group of substances that are naturally soluble in an alcohol water solution. First an extract of the

source material is obtained by soaking the ground or macerated material in alcohol for specified periods to obtain the
first solution known as a *mother tincture*. In some instances the
whole plant may be immersed and used in the production of
the medicines, or in others particular parts such as the leaves,
roots, flowers, seed or berries are employed, or perhaps a combination of these parts, as laid down in the *Homoeopathic Pharmacopoeia*.

The precise details in the methods of handling specimens
vary for different plants. As a general rule a fresh plant, with a
moderately high water content, such as *Calendula officinalis* –
marigold, or *Euphrasia* - eyebright, is gently washed to remove
dust, etc., macerated in a mincer, soaked in pure alcohol for
several days then filtered to produce the mother tincture, or
first solution. But with other plants the water content is first
reduced by hanging the plant up for a few days before soaking
it to prepare the mother tincture. With specimens such as
bark or dried seeds that are already relatively dry, the mother
tincture is prepared by soaking them for a longer period in an
alcohol-water solution prior to filtering. Whichever method is
used the aim is to obtain, after filtering, a solution which can
then either be stored, or used for producing the extracts of the
original plant that will be prescribed in homoeopathic treatment. Such a mother tincture can be the starting point for
potentization.

What then is 'potentization'? It is the method used to
obtain the variously small extracts of, for instance, a plant
remedy, widely prescribed in homoeopathy. The dilutions are
a serial progression on 1:10 or 1:100 series. The sequence
followed is signified by the appropriate Latin numeral, so that
the 1:10 is referred to as the decimal, or *x* series, the 1:100 as
the centesimal, or *c* series. There are additional letters from
some Continental sources where the 1:10 series may be
referred to as *D* potencies and the 1:100 as the *CH*, centesimal
Hahnemann. In the United States the most commonly used
potencies are the decimal, or *x* series.

Succussion

That is an introduction to the terminology: now for a summary of the production. On the *x* series one drop of the mother tincture is mixed with nine drops of alcohol to give a 1:10 solution. This is then vigorously shaken with impact on a hard surface for a specific length of time, a process known technically in homoeopathy as *succussion*. This gives a *1x* potency, the first stage in the *x* series. One drop of this added to another nine drops of alcohol and vigorously shaken, gives the second stage of the *x* series, the *2x*. This will be a 1:100 dilution of the mother tincture. The series continues in this way with another dilution and succussion at each stage. A preparation commonly used is a *6x*. This will be the 1:10 series of potentization carried out six times, with dilution and succession at each stage, to give a 1:1,000,000 dilution of the mother tincture. It is important to remember that a *single* dilution of the mother tincture to 1:1,000,000 is quite different from a homoeopathic potency of *6x* which requires *six* serial dilutions and succussions.

The *c* series is prepared in a similar manner, but here the amount of diluting alcohol added is ninety-nine drops at each stage so that the dilution factor is 1:100. It means that a *2c* potency will be one part of mother tincture to ten thousand of diluent, and a *6c* one part to a million million. That is two noughts added twice for a *2c* or 1:10,000 and two noughts added six times for a *6c* or one in a million million dilution. The figures rapidly include long series of noughts. A preparation commonly used by Hahnemann and still widely employed to-day is a *30c*. This implies a dilution factor of one part with sixty noughts after it. This is two noughts added thirty times. Dilutions as fine as this are not the limit of homoeopathic potencies. A *200c* preparation or the *1000c* which is also known as *1M*, are often used. In the United States the potencies most commonly used to-day are the decimal, particularly *3x*, *6x*, *12x*, and *30x*. Of the centesimal potencies, the lower dilutions are most commonly employed, for example *6c*, *12c*, and *30c*.

Most of these dilution levels are presenting extracts beyond the stage where theoretically any original molecules should be defined as present, and this has led to some people asserting that there can be no active ingredient left in the highly dilute potencies. Such suggestions are opposed by the clinical experience of patients, prescribers and other researchers who continue to confirm the efficacy of homoeopathy and Hahnemann's pioneer work. The dilutions may be vast, and no defined molecules be detectable, but there is a large and increasing area of experience that today endorses their effects in plants, animals, children and adults. It is unfortunate if the subject is dismissed because at this stage of human evolution its processes are not easily understood. It is far more use if, like Hahnemann, we note an effect and try to understand it.

Having looked briefly at the preparation of potencies from substances naturally soluble in alcohol, we will move on to consider those not soluble in this way. Here again the method used today is a development of Hahnemann's original research work. His own writings and accounts from his biographies indicate the thoroughness with which he pursued this work. His standards were high. He insisted that each successive potency was prepared in fresh glassware and that each succussion should consist of 100 strokes brought firmly on to a resistant surface such as leather. (*Organon*, paragraph 270). As this was before the advent of mechanical aids, and much of Hahnemann's work was done with *30c* potencies, it must have required considerable effort from him and his colleagues.

Trituration
For the development of potentization of substances naturally insoluble in alcohol Hahnemann utilized his training as a chemist. He discovered that grinding such substances as mercury, calcium carbonate or sulphur with powdered sugar of milk eventually changed them to a form that could be dissolved in alcohol. He gave precise instructions about his

original method advocating grinding, for instance, one grain of mercury with 100 grains of milk sugar, taking one part of this to another 100 grains of the diluent and then repeating the process a third time to produce the 1:1,000,000 extraction or the *3c* potency, a 'solid potency'. He said that the process should take about three hours. He found that this produced an extract of mercury soluble in alcohol so that further potencies could then be made using the method advised for agents naturally soluble in this diluent, or 'liquid potencies'. It was clearly an arduous process, carefully developed and recorded. For such a repetitive grinding to produce an alcohol-soluble extract Hahnemann used the term 'trituration'. The word is still used today to refer to this process. The amount of trituration required varies with different agents but the essential aim is always to achieve intimate mixing. Although most become alcohol soluble at the *3c* stage, some of them require more than this. Silica, for instance, only becomes soluble at *5c* or *6c*, that is the fifth or sixth trituration of one part of the extract with ninety-nine parts of milk sugar.

The cardinal features of Hahnemann's methods for preparing potencies both of the naturally alcohol-water soluble substances, and those that are insoluble are still employed today in the production of homoeopathic medicines. The precise methods have of course been updated to facilitate the work. But they still employ the principles discovered and recorded by Hahnemann. To-day some manufacturers have the succussion between each serial dilution performed by hand, some allow for machines to do this part of the work. But whichever method is used, it is continuing the serial dilution and succussion pioneered by Hahnemann.

Each stage in the manufacture of homeopathic medicines to-day is rigorously controlled, not only according to the standards set by Hahnemann and his successors, but by contemporary legal controls. Fortunately, so far at least, these have not impeded the manufacture of the highly rarified dilutions of medicines widely prescribed in homoeopathy.

Dispensing of Homoeopathic Potencies

The processes discussed so far give a liquid preparation with the extract of the original agent dissolved in alcohol. Many readers will already have discovered that today a large number, if not most homoeopathic medicines, are in the form of pillules or tablets, and they may be wondering how these are produced. It is simply that to facilitate the dispensing a certain number of drops of the liquid extraction are added to plain lactose pillules or tablets which then act as carriers for the potency. With vigorous shaking the drops added to the bottle of tablets or pillules become distributed throughout their bulk so that each tablet or pillule is impregnated with some of the original solution. An alternative carrier widely used in recent years has been lactose powder. Many patients, and especially infants, became accustomed to shaking, or having shaken for them, a small amount of medicated powder onto their tongue from a piece of paper into which a single dose had been folded.

In addition to pillules, tablets or powders, homoeopathic medicines have often been dispensed as drops. With this presentation the extract is carried in a dilute alcohol solution. The drops can be a particularly easy method of giving homoeopathic medicines to young children and animals.

There are of course many other routes by which medicines are commonly taken today. Examples are the use of creams; eye, nose or ear drops; suppositories and injection. Occasionally homoeopathic medicines can also be given by non-oral routes, but this is far less common than with orthodox medication. Homoeopathic medicines are fairly often prescribed in creams or ointments, but other routes of administration are the exception rather than the rule. An example of a cream widely used in homoeopathy is *Calendula*. It contains extracts from the marigold. Examples of its usefulness are seen with certain kinds of eczema or for minor injuries. Many people have found it a useful addition to a first aid kit.

A large number of the medicines prescribed in homoeopathy have been in frequent use for many decades. A major part of the *Materia Medica* was investigated first for homoeopathic use by Hahnemann, his family and the colleagues who joined him early in the development of the practice and helped carry out the provings of the medicines. Over the years since those initial studies new data have been added and the understanding of how to prescribe them has increased. In addition to adding new data on already known medicines, homoeopaths and interested friends have continued to research new remedies. These, too, have been added to reference books to give more guides for prescribing. We referred earlier to the use of potencies of penicillin that can at times assist in the treatment of side-effects from this antibiotic or for similar effects occurring from other causes. As penicillin was only discovered in the 1940's the extract used in homoeopathy is a relatively recent addition to the prescribing manuals. Relative, that is, to medicines researched by Hahnemann. The basic idea of the *similia* principle on which homoeopathy is founded clearly leads to endless possibilities for research into new homoeopathic medicines.

Any branch of medicine, or indeed any other study, needs constantly to be researching its present practices, gaining new insights into these and finding new methods of developing them. The alternative would be a stagnant repetition with practices becoming increasingly out of date. The application of this principle in homoeopathy had led to constant searching, both for a greater understanding of the medicines already in use, and for new ones. We referred earlier to the provings carried out by Hahnemann in the early development of homoeopathy. Such tests to investigate the effects of medicinal agents on healthy people have continued throughout the decades following his work and are still pursued today. They are an important means of adding to the prescribing data for homoeopathic medicine.

As provings have been of such importance both for the early

development and continuing practice of homoeopathy, they will be considered in more detail in the next chapter.

Chapter 4

Provings

The present practice of homoeopathy began with a proving when Hahnemann demonstrated to his own satisfaction that china, an extract of Peruvian bark, could produce in his own healthy person symptoms similar to those they could treat in a patient suffering from malaria. That was in 1791. The use of provings to disclose medicines capable of helping with the treatment of a wide range of diseases has continued since then.

An earlier chapter contained a brief reference to Hahnemann's ideas and instructions concerning provings, the aim now is to take a closer look at them.

The German word of which proving is a translation was coined by Hahnemann to refer to the experiments in which a physician observed, either in himself or in volunteers, the effects of specified medicines. The aim was to take a dose large enough and for a sufficient length of time to produce clinical effects; yet small enough to be safe. Whilst taking the agent under test, the 'prover', that is the person having the medicine, reported in detail the effects occurring.

Such provings are an obvious application of the *similia* principle stating that an agent can treat symptoms occurring in a disease that are similar to effects it can induce in a healthy person. It means that prescribing data can be obtained by testing new agents to see what effects they cause in healthy volunteers who take them.

A fundamental aim often stated by Hahnemann was to test medicines away from the scene of obvious disease. As he pointed out, disease commonly provokes anxiety, as well as many other emotions, that can make it very difficult to form a clear assessment in a sickroom of a patient's response to treatment. We will all be familiar with the way in which a natural fear of disease and death can affect not only the patient and his assessment of what is happening to him, but also the opinions of those seeking to help. The avoidance of such hazards was one of the reasons that Hahnemann stated to support the use of provings by healthy people. Obviously the understanding of medicines and their effects were also observed in treatment situations. But from the beginnings of contemporary homoeopathy such reports were not the primary source of information for subsequent prescribing. Provings on healthy volunteers were to meet this need.

In theory such testing sounds simple. In practice it is often difficult. Hahnemann's instructions to provers show that he was aware that many factors other than the intrinsic power of the remedy could influence the findings of such test procedures. A summary of these instructions can be found in paragraphs 122 – 142 of the sixth edition of the *Organon*. He advises, for instance, taking only one agent at a time and avoiding food or drink that could have a stimulant or other medicinal effect. He even asks that the prover:

. . . avoid all over-exertion of mind and body, all sorts of dissipation and any disturbing passions, he should have no urgent business to distract his attention, he must devote himself to careful self-observation and not be disturbed whilst so engaged, his body must be in what is for him a good state of health, and he must possess a sufficient amount of intelligence to be able to express and describe his sensations in accurate terms.

In another paragraph he advised that the diet of provers should be simple but nourishing and exclude spices, green vegetables, salads, herb soups and stimulating drinks. His standards were high.

Today when provings are carried out they are still intended as far as possible to comply with Hahnemann's requirements. But this is often difficult with the tempo of life today, as well as the widely acknowledged influences of fertilizers, or other chemical additives on plants and animal products. It is clearly difficult to comply strictly with Hahnemann's advice on the procedure for provings. However, it could be argued that since the recipients of homoeopathy are likely to experience the effects of such factors, it is appropriate for provers to be subject to them when testing the medicines. The effect in the prover can then allow for the similar effect occurring in a patient.

How then are provings conducted today? A method widely used is for a group of provers to take a potentized medicine for several days or weeks and record the effects. The prover is asked to note any change that he observes in his physical, emotional or thought processes. The records may be in a diary form with the prover making a note each day of any changes in his health that he thinks are different from his normal pattern. Alternatively the provers are asked to complete questionnaires with selected questions about particular body functions. In addition, provers are usually asked to make regular contact with a doctor or another practitioner organizing the proving so that their reports can be checked and if necessary be clarified. As observed earlier, the aim is to take the agent being tested for long enough to disclose its effect in a healthy person. In someone not showing symptoms likely to be treated by the agent concerned it usually takes several weeks to obtain reports of its action. Occasionally, however, for instance in highly sensitive individuals, changes occur quickly. If that happens, and the prover prefers to stop them, they simply cease taking the substance being tested. The effect of such a minute dose then clears, usually very quickly.

Placebo Effects

A comment is needed here on placebo effects, or responses due more to an expectation of what a medicine may provoke than to its biological action. It was noted briefly in a previous chapter that a placebo effect had not been acknowledged in the time of Hahnemann and that it would therefore be inappropriate to criticize him for making no reference to it in his discussions of provings. Today, however, such an effect is widely observed and due account of it has to be taken in testing homoeopathic medicines. Various methods have been discussed as ways of reducing the bias placebo effect is likely to cause in any therapeutic test.

One method is for 50 per cent of provers to have an active remedy and 50 per cent a placebo, with the distribution pattern unknown to them. As a further safeguard the precise distribution is also unknown by the person giving out the test agent. The unnamed preparations can be coded for instance by number, and the code known only to a third party. Such a precaution has at times been increased by giving a placebo to all participants without their knowledge of it, for the first few days or weeks of a trial with the 50:50 allocation of placebo : active remedy being given subsequently. It has been suggested that such a precaution further reduces the distortion of results that could easily arise in the early stages of a proving when an associated anxiety or uncertainty is likely to be highest.

Another method of reducing placebo bias is to do very extensive provings and accept as signs of a medicinal effect only those changes that occur in a significant proportion of the group.

It is as important to observe and allow for the placebo effect as it is difficult to prevent its bias of results. An allowance needs to be made for it in all medical tests with patients or healthy volunteers. It applies both to conventional and homoeopathic medicine and concerns observations of responses to prescriptions given for a disease process as well as tests planned as experiments with healthy people.

Toxicology

Although such provings are an important source of data for prescribing homoeopathic medicine, they are not the only one. The *similia* principle can also be applied in other ways for researching new remedies. Another clear example of the application of the principle occurs when prescribing data are obtained from toxicology studies. The reported effects of poisonings give data that, according to the *similia* principle, can become a guide for prescribing a homoeopathic medicine for diseases which, although from a different source, mimic the described toxic effects. An earlier chapter referred briefly to this with mention of the way in which reports of the toxic effects of mercury and arsenic could yield prescribing data for these two substances. There are many other examples. A large number of the medicines used in a very dilute form in homoeopathic provings and practice would be highly toxic in their crude state. Hence reports of accidental poisonings can be further aids to building up an understanding of the symptoms for which a particular medicine may be appropriate.

A particular example of such a use of reports from accidental poisonings occurred with the initial studies by a homoeopathic doctor of a preparation since widely known as *Lachesis*. The story is reported in *Guiding Symptoms*, Volume VI, by Herring, one of the pioneer homoeopaths. It tells, how, in 1828, he was on a botanical expedition to the Upper Amazon with his wife, accompanied by some natives from the area. He had been told about the dreaded Surukuku snake, but still insisted that he wanted one for research. To improve his chances of getting one he offered a reward for a live specimen and eventually one was brought to him. It is reported that the terrified natives fled, leaving Herring handling the snake alone. He stunned the snake, held its head with a forked stick then expressed the venom onto milk sugar. Even handling the venom and preparing low potencies from it brought about in Herring a fever, excitement and delerium. Later, it is reported, he slept, then on waking he first demanded a drink and then asked what he had done and said. The account was written down and became the first proving of *Lachesis*. Later the natives gradually returned and were astonished to find Herring still alive.

The account of this episode illustrates the way in which accidental poisonings can contribute to prescribing data. It also shows the dedication of the pioneer homoeopaths. Fortunately, not all provings need involve such risks! Most of the subsequent provings of *Lachesis* were done with a *30c* potency or, an even higher degree of potentization.

From such provings a picture was gradually compiled of effects that include chest constriction, dizziness and severe ringing in the ears, a worsening of symptoms on waking from sleep, throat pain, bruising and haemorrhages. Applying such data *Lachesis* has since been widely and effectively used in appropriate potencies in conditions as various as asthma, Ménières disease and menopausal symptoms.

Materia Medica and Repertories

From a combination of reports from provings and toxicology, descriptions were gradually formed of many clinical conditions that could be produced by the agents named. Over the years the reports were collected and gradually accumulated into prescribing manuals known as '*Materia Medica*'. The name implies that they attempt to present systematic reviews of the reported effects and therefore prescribing indications for homoeopathic medicines. There are many such books. The particularly well-known ones include those by Dr J.T. Kent, an American homoeopathic doctor who practised in the early nineteenth century, Dr J.H. Clarke, a British homoeopathic doctor who practised in the early twentieth century, Constantine Herring referred to in the description of the early *Lachesis* proving, and Hughes. These are all major reference works. Smaller summaries of the *Materia Medica* have been written by other homoeopaths. Well-known ones include those by Boericke and Allen. A short but practical and helpful introduction to the *Materia Medica* can be found in *Introduction to Homoeopathic Medicine* by Dr H. Boyd, published in 1981 by Keats Publishing Inc. Another recent publication has been a review of the Materia Medica written in 1980 by Jouanny, a French homoeopathic doctor. Another French homoeopathic doctor has also contributed a major book containing reports on recent provings. This is *Materia Medica of New Homoeopathic Remedies* by Dr O.A. Julian, published in English in 1979 by Beaconsfield Press and in America by Keats Publishing Inc.

In such *Materia Medica* the individual medicines are listed, usually alphabetically, and accounts given of the effects each one can provoke or treat. Another set of prescribing manuals present the data the other way round. They start with named symptoms and give remedies previously found appropriate to their treatment. These are called 'repertories'. There are many of them in the homoeopathic libraries.

A more recent method of presenting homoeopathic prescribing data had developed with the advent of computers. As in other branches of medicine, there have been many discussions about how computer technology could assist its practice. Various groups are now programming computers, or have already done so, to present when required appropriate summaries of prescribing data.

Clearly all such accounts, whether they are *Materia Medica*, repertories or computer print-outs are merely aids to prescribings. They are not directives. The books and computer print-outs usefully present reports on effects of homoeopathic remedies. But the process of prescribing will always require far more than reference to such records. As Dr J.H. Clarke says in the introduction to his *Materia Medica* – 'Homoeopathy is the art of individualizing'. He reminds his readers that prescribing has to refer to individual needs presented now. And although prescribers can refer to reports of earlier provings and prescribing experiences they have to re-assess these in relation to the present requirements. Many writers have reminded us that as the situation in which we live and work is constantly changing, so too are the signs of disease and the prescriptions appropriate to help treat them. Data from past investigations are clearly an aid but there is constantly the need to revise and update them. Consequently, not even a computer programmed with all the available data from *Materia Medica* or repertories could give a necessarily definitive answer for a disease-state presenting now.

In assessing provings and using them to assist prescribing there is therefore a two-fold need. On the one hand we need to clarify the insights previously expressed. That is, we need to work on the ideas that have already emerged and proved helpful to our health and development, seeking for clarification of their details and implications. At the same time, and paradoxically, we need to be ready to change the insights given as new situations and insights develop. Provings are not dogma. They are partial reports on the effects of certain agents recorded at a specific moment in time. As we change, our provings will also change. Behaviour patterns and reactions of people have obviously altered since provings were first done nearly 200 years ago. Our *Materia Medica* will therefore always need revising and extending. It is paradoxical that we need to go on using our prescribing data, yet in a constant readiness to modify them.

In the next chapter we will consider how we can apply such insights for homoeopathic prescribing today.

Chapter 5

Homoeopathic Prescribing Today

As Hahnemann said nearly two hundred years ago, there are three stages in the understanding and practice of medicine, a knowledge of disease, a knowledge of the medicines that can treat it and how to put these two together. This chapter considers the third stage in this triad. The first stage was discussed mainly in Chapter 1 in conjunction with the *similia* principle. It referred to the idea that disease is a product of changes in psychological as well as physical energies, and that it can be corrected by a medicine capable of provoking similar symptoms in a healthy person. The second stage, a knowledge of medicines was the main subject of Chapters 3 and 4. They referred to the methods used to discover sources of medicines and to prepare from them the extracts, or potencies, able to help treat disease. The discussion also referred to some ideas concerning the nature of potentized medicines. The third stage is the practical application of such ideas in therapy. It is an examination of how a homoeopathic prescriber decides on a medicine, its strength and its frequency, for a particular patient.

In essence, the aim is simply to match the learning obtained about effects medicines can produce with the symptoms seen in a disease. Several times in earlier chapters there have been references to the attempt in homoeopathic prescribing to understand as much as we can about the person experiencing the disease as well as the particular symptoms of which they now complain. This is all part of the symptom picture to be taken into account for homoeopathic prescribing. Because of this it is often said that homoeopathy treats the 'whole person'. But there is a need for caution about such claims. Human understanding is only slowly developing, and we do not know what constitutes the 'whole person'. It is therefore more precise to say that homoeopathy aims to find a treatment appropriate to as much as can be at present understood about a person requesting treatment.

Such a comprehensive assessment of patients and their diseases implies the need for a system to classify their reports. To write down an assortment of jumbled data would be of little use. That would be like throwing the pieces of a jigsaw puzzle onto a table and hoping they fell into the picture from which they were cut. Just as the puzzle pieces need to be sorted out and fitted into a picture, similarly a system is needed for the assessment and linkage of pieces of information given when a patient reports a disease he is experiencing.

The Diagnosis
So how does a homoeopathic prescriber set about clarifying the information presented to him?

It is often said that a consultation begins as a patient comes into the room. Frequently the way in which someone walks, their tones of voice and their appearance give important clues to what they are feeling. Obviously many people put up a front and deliberately try to hide some aspects of their experience. But even this can be a point to note for later prescribing. Many homoeopathic doctors begin by inviting patients to talk about their problems in a manner similar to that used by most physicians. A homoeopathic doctor needs a review of symptoms similar to that required for any type of prescribing. But in addition to this he also requires particular details of symptoms unlikely to be pursued in other branches of medicine. This is one of the special features of homoeopathy and it will be discussed in detail after this initial summary of the process. A homoeopathic doctor will also use, where appropriate, the standard forms of physical examinations and special tests that may help towards understanding a disease.

Although such tests can be useful aids for homoeopathic prescribing they are only a small part of the data required. The larger part comes from the patients' own reports of their symptoms and their answers to questions put by the prescriber. For homoeopathic prescribing many of the questions asked may sound strange to patients who have previously known only a non-homoeopathic approach. For instance, the quality of a pain may be a factor to note for homoeopathic prescribing. A patient and his family unaccustomed to this were surprised to hear a homoeopathic doctor ask 'does the pain make you say ouch or arrhh?'. Some of the points to be clarified need detailed questioning. Others can begin as a patient enters a consulting room. As noted earlier, the way he walks, shakes hands and sits down can say a great deal about how a patient is feeling.

So how do we attempt to clarify and record the many data that can be used in homoeopathic prescribing? One method is to use a three-stage approach looking first at the particular symptoms presented now, secondly at the general reactions of a patient to his situation and thirdly at how this process has developed.

First, then, a review of the symptoms of a particular disease. Here the emphasis is placed on a specific problem such as a cough or constipation. Whatever the problem, the prescriber will require a detailed description of its nature. If it is a pain he will probably need to know its position, quality, timing and severity. Often patients seem surprised at such questions and say 'pain is pain'. But when asked further they can distinguish such types as aching, cutting or burning. If, for instance, the problem is a migraine type of headache, the prescriber will probably ask about the quality of pain, whether it is more likely to occur at particular times of day or night, whether it is eased or made worse by lying down, what effect sleep has on it, its position, how long it lasts and how frequently it occurs. If the problem is diarrhoea again a detailed description will be required clarifying as far as possible its character, timing and any associated pain, urging or blood loss. Sometimes a lot of detail is supplied and extensive further questioning may not be required. But, if need be, the prescriber will clarify the reports.

So far a non-homoeopathic doctor may well have taken a very similar account. The 'extras' of a homoeopathic approach become evident when additional or qualifying questions are asked concerning the reports already given. For instance, concerning most pains he is likely to ask, 'do they come in sudden surges, or build up and recede gradually?' Even if it is a problem not usually associated with body movement a homoeopathic doctor often asks if the symptoms are better or worse for movement. Other commonly asked qualifying questions are, 'does it vary with the time of day or night? Is it worse in a hot or cold room; worse indoors or outside?' A patient with stomach problems may be asked, not simply which foods help or hinder him, but whether their being hot or cold makes a difference. Other factors, such as effects from changes in the weather, may well be an aid for homoeopathic prescribing. These are just a few examples of the qualifying questions a homoeopathic prescriber may ask concerning a patient's primary symptoms.

So far, we have focused on what a patient probably regards as 'his disease'. The second stage in this three-part approach concerns the associated general reactions of a patient, what he is more inclined to describe as 'I myself'. For instance, a patient may say 'my knee is worse in cold weather, but I feel better for it', distinguishing his general response from effects on a particular symptom. It is the stage in taking the account of a disease process where the attention is turned to focus on the mood, thought processes and general interests and reactions of a patient, and any changes shown in these since the disease has developed. The information requested may concern the responses of an individual patient to weather conditions, room temperature, time of day, various foods and drinks, being indoors or outside, being in sea or mountain air and being in company or alone. It covers a wide range. But let it be emphasized again, it is concerned with the response of the person generally, rather than how his particular symptoms react to such factors. At times patients say, 'I feel better in myself in sea air, or in a cold room, but my throat, (or whatever else the local complaint may be,) feels worse there'. All of this can be taken into account for homoeopathic prescribing. In addition to this some homoeopathic prescribers attach importance to body build, hair and eye colour. These too are said by some prescribers to help in selecting an appropriate medicine.

Closely related to such a general review of a patient is an appraisal of how a disease has influenced his interests and thought processes. Some people readily admit that disease such as a sore throat can provoke depression and negative gloomy thoughts. Other reactions include irritability, anxiety or even at times aggressive behaviour. This sort of reaction is well-known. Other people with illness may become more placid than is their norm. The varieties of response are vast, and can be important guides for homoeopathic prescribing.

It sometimes happens that while a patient gives an account of their particular complaints, their general reactions to them become obvious. Adults often show many of their reactions in their tone of voice. Children usually do it more strongly by action as well as voice. For example, two sisters with hay fever were brought to see a homoeopathic doctor. Both had similar problems in the summer with streaming noses and eyes after exposure to grass pollen. The older sister was tall, thin, shy and reluctant to discuss her symptoms. The six-year old smiled coyly at everyone, delighted in being questioned and appeared thoroughly to enjoy coming for a medical examination. Although their hay fever symptoms were remarkably similar, the two girls received different prescriptions.

The third stage in this form of homoeopathic assessment is concerned with a detailed and far-ranging review of how these effects have developed. Often patients can readily describe when and where recent pains or other symptoms started, and how they have changed. At times, however, questions are needed to jog their memories, especially if symptoms have been present for a long time. The account of how a patient's illness has developed is usually an important part of any medical assessment. But as with the review of symptoms, homoeopathic prescribers are likely to add to it some extra lines of questioning that can be additional guides for this form of treatment. Any doctor asking a patient about a disease will probably ask how it started and developed. But homoeopathic prescribers are likely to take note of associations that would not appear important for non-homoeopathic treatment. If symptoms develop after an acute infection, or severe shock, even though to ordinary medical thought they may appear unrelated this may be highly significant for homoeopathic prescribing. For instance, a child or adult may develop recurrent stomach symptoms for which no clear cause can be found. If, on listening to the patient, a homoeopathic prescriber found that these upsets followed an infection such as measles or influenza he would probably prescribe the homoeopathic treatment for that earlier disease even though in ordinary medical thought stomach upsets are not usually attributed to it.

Similarly, if diseases presenting now are traced by a patient back to the effects of a vaccination or an accident a homoeopath may well prescribe treatment appropriate to the earlier disturbance even though in conventional medical practice the two may not usually be linked. An example of this occurred recently when a patient with widespread dermatitis requested homoeopathic treatment. She was given a prescription but at first the symptoms did not improve. After going over her story again she remembered that the skin problem developed shortly after she reacted strongly against a smallpox vaccination. Her homoeopathic treatment was changed to a prescription often advised for adverse effects of such vaccine and her skin steadily improved.

Closely related to this form of questioning about the symptoms a patient presents is a review of their family history. Homoeopathic prescribers often take note of major illnesses experienced by close relatives. Even though the reports usually concern diseases that are not regarded as hereditary, a note about when they occurred can help towards a clearer understanding of how a person has developed and which homoeopathic medicines may help him now. In many homoeopathic books frequent reference is made to 'miasms', or ancestral disease patterns, which are said to influence a patient now even though he shows no evidence of the physical expression of the particular disease. Many homoeopathic prescribers aim to treat such hereditary traits. It is an interesting theory which continues to be extensively discussed in homoeopathic literature.

Taking such a detailed account of a patient's reports of disease implies the need for a scheme in writing notes. The three-stage approach suggested here is just one of many that can be used. In many homoeopathic books the symptoms are listed according to the different parts of the body, starting with the head and mind and working through to the limbs. This form of presentation is widely used in books summarizing data for prescribing.

Another system frequently used in homoeopathy was devised by Dr J.T. Kent, an American homoeopath practising around the beginning of this century. Its terminology may therefore sound old-fashioned but it is appropriate to include it here as it is still widely applied and usefully reminds us of the areas to examine when taking a homoeopathic history. Kent suggested that the account of symptoms should be referred to three areas. He called them 'mentals, generals and particulars'. He placed 'mentals' first as he suggested that such inner responses were of particular, or even prime, importance in assessing a disease process. Responses to be assessed here included thought processes, interests of an individual, whether they were inclined to mix readily with other people, or preferred to be solitary and whether they were organized or untidy, determined or yielding. Kent suggested that such traits gave strong leads towards indicating the will of an individual, their prime determinant, and were therefore very important in selecting a remedy likely to help them. Assessments of such *inner* 'mental' or private concerns were first in Kent's approach to homoeopathic prescribing and were followed by a look at 'general' responses, the reactions shown by patients *outwardly* to their environment. Here he included the reactions of the person as an individual to weather conditions, time of day, being in or outside, in sea air or mountains, likes or dislikes of certain foods, a preference for being quiet and resting or busy and energetic, to name but a few of the types of questioning used here. These reports concerned the reaction of the person in general, hence the term used for them, rather than the response of their particular symptoms. For instance, if a patient says 'I feel better in sea air' that is a general symptom in Kent's classification. If they also add 'but my eczema gets worse in that situation' that would come into the 'particular', his third group.

These, he suggested, were the descriptions of the local evidence of a disease. Another example would be the details about a sore throat and what soothes or aggravates it. After noting such particulars Kent referred to a fourth group of symptoms that he called 'peculiar effects', that is, changes that would be unusual for a specific disease, like perhaps, sweating heavily with a fever but not being thirsty. This assessment according to 'mentals, generals and particulars' is still widely quoted and used today. It is a useful reminder of the need, not merely to look at the particular symptoms of which someone complains, but to attempt to understand their deeper associations and perhaps even their causes.

Other Tests

As noted earlier in this chapter, a homoeopathic doctor may well augment such a detailed review of symptoms by appropriate tests such as blood or X-ray examinations. The role of such investigations in homoeopathic prescribing warrants further discussion as there has at times been an assumption that such tests are inappropriate for this form of medicine. Such assumptions may be related to particular interpretations of Hahnemann's insistence that the symptoms described by a patient, especially when they are closely questioned by a trained examiner, are the total evidence of a disease. In his writings Hahnemann says many times that the symptoms presented by a patient are the visible evidence of unseen changes in body energies that cause disease to occur. Therefore, he deduces, a *thorough* review of symptoms will give all the information needed to assess and prescribe for a particular patient.

Hahnemann was writing in the early 1800s before the advent of such investigations as blood tests and X-ray photographs that today may play an important part in helping towards an understanding of disease. The use of appropriate modern aids does not necessarily imply a rejection of Hahnemann's views. Hahnemann's concern was to get an insight into forces operating in the body to produce the gross symptoms of diseases. His assertion that symptoms of diseases are outward signs of inner changes are as valid today as in his time and can be applied as much to the reports of images produced by X-rays or blood cells, as to verbal descriptions of, for instance, a persistent cough and tight chest. Even with the refined tests of disease widely used today, Hahnemann's questioning and opinions are valid. It is frequently observed in medicine today that the more we learn, the more we realize there is to learn. The data from special tests are still describing effects of disease that Hahnemann may well have called outward 'symptoms' rather than inner causes. Such findings therefore still invite questioning of their cause. Hence it may be argued that when homoeopathic doctors today use appropriate special tests, and question their findings as Hahnemann advised, that they are extending his work rather than conflicting with it.

Three-Part Man

The comprehensive assessment of symptoms strongly advised by Hahnemann and developed later by Kent and other homoeopaths compares closely with an approach often advised in medicine generally today that looks at human function, in health or disease, in relation to 'three-part man'. There was reference to this in an earlier chapter. It is appropriate to include it again now as it is a particularly useful way of thinking about the processes that operate within us and can be another guide for building up the assessment for homoeopathic prescribing.

Physically we need a head, chest and abdomen. Human functions can continue without arms or legs but the three zones of head, chest and abdomen are essential to proper organic function. These three zones can be related to the three aspects of thought, emotion and appetival drive. The head and brain represent cognition and reasoning; the chest, with the heart and lungs symbolizes the feeling life, affections, emotional assessments and responses; the abdomen, with the emphasis on organs specialized for handling food and sex, is a focus for appetival drive.

Hence the three basic anatomical zones represent the three basic psychological activities of man, namely the ability to pursue a course of action, feel its effects and think about the process. The symbology reminds us that just as healthy physical function requires the interaction of the three zones, similarly psychological health occurs when there is a correct balance of drive to act, awareness of its effects and definition of the process. It is a linkage in a single act of firm decision, sensitive feeling and clear reason. One way of building up a picture of a disease process is to question its effects on these three aspects of a person's activities. As a further step this three part assessment can be applied in considering how homoeopathic medicines work. One way of approaching this question is to say that a correct *similia* suited to all of the three sections it names can help towards their integration, that is, towards fitting them into a better balance and therefore aiding a return to health.

As so often happens, different systems for classifying sections of a subject in practice become similar to each other. Such a similarity can be seen in Kent's system for taking a homoeopathic patient's history and the three-part man assessment. The 'mentals' to which Kent referred can be compared to the intellect or thought processes. Kent used the term 'generals' to refer to the responses of an individual to his environment. They can be compared to the liking or disliking reactions that today are usually referred to as emotional responses. The 'particulars' described by Kent referred to the physical symptoms and are comparable to the physical drive with its focus on the gross aspects of human function. Both systems are useful reminders of the need to watch for the ways in which thoughts and feelings influence all our physical activities.

To people familiar with homoeopathy the classification used by Kent will probably be well-known and may be their preferred method for assessing symptoms. To others the terms used by Kent may appear out of date and an alternative system be preferred. The three-part man view is one such alternative. Whichever system is used it is an aid to clarifying the data given when we are trying to understand someone's report of disease. It can also remind us about the aspects we need to consider in talking with a patient, or in assessing our own needs.

Clearly to take such a detailed review of symptoms from a

patient is not always possible. It may be ideal to prescribe from a detailed review of all available data presented in this three-fold manner. But we do not live in an ideal world and such a full assessment is not always possible. Homoeopathic prescribers often have to learn to work fast and may at times need to base their prescription on a report of symptoms that has focused mainly on the particular physical complaints.

Pathological Prescribing

Over the years since Hahnemann began developing the present practice of homoeopathic medicine a method of prescribing has developed which tends to emphasize the local physical effects of disease. It is known as 'pathological prescribing'. The selection of a prescription by this method still applies the *similia* principle, but instead of paying a lot of attention to the more general aspects of a disease process, it refers particularly to the specific physical complaints. It means for instance that if someone asks for a homoeopathic medicine to help with tennis elbow, a remedy such as *Ruta* may be prescribed without first asking a lot of questions about which conditions at present make the patient feel generally better or worse. Such 'pathological' prescribing is particularly useful in first aid. A common example is the use of homoeopathic extracts of *Arnica*. An extract of this plant has helped many people with bruising or shock after injury, whatever their general likes and dislikes or thought processes have been.

Constitutional Prescribing

Such pathological prescribing contrasts the approach that aims to use a full account of symptoms, known technically as 'constitutional' prescribing. Dr Kent introduced this term as a reminder that homoeopathic prescribing was to be based, in his view, on a review of the whole constitution of the patient, as far as this could be assessed. He did not advocate pathological prescribing. It has sometimes been thought that

Hahnemann advised 'constitutional' prescribing. Although Hahnemann recommended prescribing on the whole picture as far as possible, the term constitutional was not introduced by him. That word came in later with the work of Kent.

Today both systems are widely used, often together. It is possible for instance to prescribe one remedy that appears to suit the general temperament or psychological state of a person as well as their particular symptoms, and shortly after this another one with special emphasis on a particular physical problem they are experiencing. For instance, a lady who recently asked for homoeopathic medicine after surgery to her foot also had multiple sclerosis. The prescription recommended for her included a 'constitutional' remedy to help her generally, and a pathological one to help with the healing of her foot.

Even when there is an emphasis on apparently localized symptoms, it is still possible to be watchful for signs of the general response to them shown by a patient. Another example may help clarify this point. Two women report that they are troubled by cystitis. They may both have similar symptoms as regards frequency of passing urine, with pain in the process and occasional blood in it. They may even have similar results from a specimen sent to a laboratory for analysis. But it can quickly be observed in talking to them that one of them is chilly, sweating moderately, reluctant to talk about her problems, wants sympathy from no one, and has only come for advice because her symptoms are a sufficient nuisance to make her ask for help. The other woman is very different in manner. Clearly she is very ready to ask for help. She is easy-going, enjoys sympathy and hopes, though she may not say so, that the cystitis will provoke for her some increased signs of compassion and affection from her family. Both women may have similar bladder problems, but their reactions to them are very different. In homoeopathic practice different medicines would be indicated for them. Although the discussion of symptoms may be brief and focused on the bladder difficulties, many other reactions can also be easily assessed and used in prescribing.

Choice of Potency

The selection of the remedy required is only the first step in prescribing. The second one is to decide on the potency, that is the degree of dilution and succussion of the medicine. After this it only remains to advise on the frequency and when to take it.

Over the years since Hahnemann began developing the present-day practice of homoeopathy there has been considerable debate about which potency should be used and when. Some homoeopathic prescribers have strong views favouring either a 'high' or 'low' potency. Most use varying potencies, depending on the diseases being treated. Some of these terms have been introduced in an earlier chapter, but as many of them may be unfamiliar to readers it may be helpful again to summarize their implications. *Potentization* is the process of serial dilution and succussion, that is a rhythmic shaking with impact, by which a homoeopathic medicine is prepared. The potency is the strength of the product. The *c* or centesimal scale implies dilution and succussion on the 1:100 series, the *x* or *D* scale the 1:10 series. A potency of less than *30c* is usually termed *low*. Those of *30c* and over are termed *high*. This means that *6c* is a *low* potency, *200c* is *high*. In general many homoeopathic prescribers advise short courses of a high potency for acute disease, long courses of a low potency for chronic disease. Let it be said immediately that this is not a rule, it is only a general guide, a practice widely used but by no means a definite line to follow. There are more terms here that may need clarifying. The words 'acute' and 'chronic' here refer to the length of time for which a disease has existed. In medical practice a disease of short duration, such as a few hours or days is usually termed acute. One lasting many weeks, months or even years, is termed chronic.

In homoeopathic practice common examples of prescribing

are a *30c* medicine several times for one or two days in acute disease. Whereas, for chronic disease the pattern is more likely to be a *6c* medicine two or three times daily for several days or even a few weeks. A useful guide is to advise stopping the remedy as soon as the symptoms improve. With acute disease hopefully that will be in a day or two. If an improvement is not occurring in this time the prescription probably needs changing. For some chronic diseases it may be necessary to continue a prescription after a partial improvement has occurred. A common example is chronic arthritis. For this complaint or for other longer-lasting disorders, patients often need to go on taking their homoeopathic medicines for a long time in order to establish an easing of the symptoms.

Another very practical question is how are the medicines taken. An earlier chapter referred to their presentation in liquid, powder or tablet form. Probably to-day in the U.S., tablets are most widely used. Many homoeopaths have followed Hahnemann's advice that tablets should be sucked slowly to enable absorption from the mouth. Taking them about half-an-hour away from food is often said further to assist absorption. Some prescribers follow Hahnemann's practice and advise avoiding coffee, tea or strong toothpaste when taking homoeopathic medicine. But there is not general agreement on this.

A very practical question today concerns the interaction between homoeopathic and other appropriate forms of medicine. Such a combination has been found to be safe in many years of practice. The question of how and when to combine homoeopathic treatment with other medication, or with other therapies, is important. It is often asked by patients seeking homoepathic help and wanting to know, for instance, would it be safe to take a non-homoeopathic type of prescription if they need to contact their General Practitioner before seeing a homoeopath again. The possibility of combining therapies is also frequently raised by doctors interested to learn of new lines of treatment that can be safely added to those they have already found helpful to patients. This important subject requires careful consideration and will occupy a major part of the next chapter.

Chapter 6

Homoeopathy –
A Complementary Therapy

For many years homoeopathy has frequently been described as one of the forms of 'alternative medicine'. This term has been widely used for several methods of treating disease; three of the particularly well-known ones being homoeopathy, acupuncture and osteopathy. In recent years there has been a change in this habit and the term 'alternative' has been widely replaced by 'complementary'. In many ways this change of description has been significant and helpful. When the word 'alternative' was applied to homoeopathy there was, at times, a tendency to assume that this meant that a patient had to choose between homoeopathic *or* other treatment. It was often thought that it was an either/or decision. Fortunately such an attitude is rarely seen today. Most patients and prescribers now using homoeopathy regard it as one of many lines of therapy which may be appropriate to help an individual. To many of us the shift away from the term 'alternative medicine' towards describing it as 'complementary' is a welcome change signifying this co-operative rather than competitive role. It implies that homoeopathy is a method of treatment that can be used in conjunction with, or as a complement to, other appropriate methods of therapy. As it is often said, it emphasizes its role as another string to the therapeutic bow.

To what then may homoeopathy be a complement? First and foremost it is a complement to the will of an individual to regain his health. This may appear to be stating the obvious but it is possible to place so much emphasis on the value of therapies applied as if from *outside* of an individual patient's own awareness and control that the faculties *within* his power are obscured. It is often observed that patients who show a healthy interest in their own therapy and do all they can to co-operate with the help offered, do better than those who anticipate difficulties in the healing process and at times even deliberately resist it. Clearly, healing requires more than interest. But the will is the prime mover of our bodies and we need to remember this whilst also acknowledging the importance of diet, appropriate medicine, other physical aids to treatment, emotional support and understanding, etc. It is as if the interest and expectation set a course with which the therapy can co-operate. Children often show this particularly clearly. A simple but common example occurs when a child makes an apparently dramatic recovery from an illness as the school day finishes and a favoured evening activity is due, or as term ends and holidays approach.

A rationale for understanding this is easier to follow is we recall again that the body in all its aspects is a complex of interacting energies. Therapy is not merely the manipulation of substantial cells, it is a realignment of all the energies co-operating to form the physical body. When the forces of the will, idea structure, emotions and their physical embodiment all co-operate with the therapy offered, there will be a combined healing effort that will clearly be more helpful than if various aspects of this system are opposing itself. It is like swimming with a steady current and going along easily rather than getting caught in conflicting streams and struggling in the process.

In considering other lines of therapy which can act in conjunction with homoeopathy the aim will again be to pursue Hahnemann's ideal as stated in the *Organon*. That is, 'to seek a return to health as speedily, gently, harmlessly and thoroughly as possible' (*Organon*, para. 2). This again may be stating the obvious, but there are occasions when patients are heard to comment that their treatment seems worse than their disease and that clearly is a situation that all therapists would wish to avoid.

Other Therapies in Conjunction with Homoeopathy

There are many forms of therapy that can be used effectively and safely in conjunction with homoeopathy. The range is vast and it will not be possible to refer to all of them here. But, hopefully, those included will illustrate the ways in which various therapies can be applied in co-operation. As is often said most, if not all, diseases have many causes and effects. Even though a disease process has a single name describing it, the associated picture usually arises from more than one cause. Hence it may well be appropriate to use various types of therapy in co-operation for the varying causal factors and their resulting symptoms.

A particularly clear illustration of the appropriateness of a combined approach occurs at times when surgery is required. The need for surgical treatment is at times clearly seen. Even though in the time of Hahnemann surgery involved more hazard and pain than are associated with the refined techniques of modern surgical and anaesthetic procedures, he advocated its appropriate use. In the *Organon*, he acknowledges that if surgery is required, homoeopathic treatment can usefully help patients before and after it. Most patients naturally feel some anxiety before an operation. Homoeopathic medicine can often help with this. When an operation is over, again homoeopathic medicine can be useful, this time to assist healing and pain reduction. *Arnica* is a homoeopathic medicine often used for this purpose, others include *Staphysagria* and *Hypericum*. Many patients have reported the beneficial effects of homoeopathic medicines prescribed in such a situation.

In acute surgical emergencies, such as a perforated stomach ulcer, the need for an operation is obvious. Similarly in orthopaedics, the need for appropriate surgical treatment may well be clear to all concerned when a patient has a complicated fracture of his leg. It has been said before that it is no use trying to set a fracture with a *10M* potency of mercury. But there are some situations where surgery is considered as a possible line of treatment in which homoeopathic medicine may help the patient and at times avert the need for an operation. An example is the early stages of gastric or duodenal ulceration. There are some types of such ulceration that may heal with appropriate diets, medicines, a reduction of cigarette smoking and other supportive measures that may reduce a stress reaction. In such situations the addition of a homoeopathic medicine has often been reported to aid the healing of an ulcer and so avert the need for surgery. When trying to help a patient with such a problem a homoeopathic doctor may well work in conjunction with a surgeon. It is just one example of many such situations where doctors from different specialities can co-operate with a patient in finding an appropriate line of treatment.

Closely allied to general surgery is obstetrics – that is medical care for pregnancy and childbirth – and its associated speciality, gynaecology, the treatment of diseases peculiar to women. In a complicated delivery, operative intervention may be essential. But in normal childbirth or even with assisted deliveries, homoeopathic medicines have often been reported to help maintain appropriate contractions of the uterus (womb) and to help reduce the amount of bleeding. For gynaecological problems needing surgery homoeopathic medicines can again assist healing. There are many other gynaecological problems not serious enough to warrant surgery, but recurrently distressing to patients, and, at times, to their families. Common examples are period pains or premenstrual tension. For problems of this sort homoeopathy may well be the only medication required to help a patient overcome such difficulties.

Homoeopathy in Infectious Diseases

When we consider medical rather than surgical problems, again homoeopathy may be used either as a complement to other forms of treatment or at times as the main line of therapy used by a patient. Homoeopathic doctors are frequently asked if they still need antibiotics for the treatment of infections or if homoeopathic medicines can avert this need. An appropriate answer to this question was given at a meeting a few months ago by a senior homoeopathic doctor now retired. She said simply, 'the more we know of homoeopathy the less we need antibiotics'. In other words, she was saying that homoeopathic treatment can sometimes, but not always, avert the need for antibiotics and the more we know about homoeopathic prescribing the less we will need to use the stronger forms of conventional medicines. For instance, patients and prescribers using homoeopathy have often found that a well-timed dose of a homoeopathic medicine can be sufficient to help them overcome an infection such as tonsillitis. An example of this occurred recently when a patient with an ulcerated throat, with the infecting organism demonstrated in a swab sent to a pathology laboratory, recovered with the help of a homoeopathic preparation of *Mercurius solubis* and without using antibiotics. Throat infections are one example of an illness where it may well be appropriate to try a homoeopathic remedy before using antibiotics.

Many homoeopathic books contain descriptions of other infections, such as bronchitis and cystitis responding to homoeopathic treatment. But we need to remember here that many of these accounts were written long before antibiotics were available. Today it is different. A wide range of antibiotics is available and homoeopathic prescribers may well need to be aware of what they have to offer. Obviously homoeopaths prefer to advise homoeopathic prescriptions, and these may well be appropriate for some kinds of infection, but at other times antibiotics may be needed. Even in this situation homoeopathic medicines may still be used for additional help. As described in an earlier chapter, at times they can also be used to reduce side-effects from antibiotics.

An example of the way in which homoeopathic medicine can help in the treatment of infection was given by a follow-up survey done at the Royal London Homoeopathic Hospital in 1976, of children referred for help with recurrent tonsillitis, ear infections, colds or catarrh. The results were assessed of children referred after needing antibiotics at least once a month for six months or once in two months for a year. They showed that of forty-five such children nearly 45 per cent had a response that, according to the mothers, was dramatic, with the children only needing antibiotics for such an infection once or less in the next six months. Another 45 per cent improved appreciably, in both severity and frequency, but not to the degree of the first group. Only 11 per cent showed little or no improvement. It is an indication of the part homoeopathic treatment can play in such recurring infection.

Arthritis
In Hahnemann's time infectious diseases were much more common than they are today. The situation has changed considerably in the last 200 years. Improvements in public health, personal hygiene, diet and medicine have contributed to this. As a result infectious diseases are not as prevalent as in former times, and other illnesses, which were less talked about in the past, now receive increasing attention. Amongst these are the various forms of arthritis. It is a particularly common complaint for which many methods of treatment can be helpful. Homoeopathy is one of them. Many patients have reported benefits from homoeopathic treatment for rheumatoid and osteo-arthritis, as well as some other less common forms of this problem.

An indication of the help homoeopathic medicine can give in the treatment of rheumatoid arthritis comes from a study done with patients attending the Glasgow Homoeopathic Hospital. This was reported in 1980 by physicians working in that unit. It showed more improvement of symptoms in patients receiving homoeopathic treatment than in a group having an inactive medicine (placebo).

Testing medicines is never easy as the results can be influenced by so many factors. It is especially difficult in homoeopathy where there is particular emphasis on prescribing for individual patients as well as taking note of the disease diagnosed by medical opinion. This makes it difficult for researchers into homoeopathy to collect a large enough sample of patients with symptoms sufficiently similar to test a single medicine in the manner often advised in conventional medical practice. However, despite this difficulty some studies have been done. The study referred to on rheumatoid arthritis is one of them and usefully illustrates the part homoeopathic medicine can play in the treatment of such disease. In general it is probably fair to say that if a disease can be helped by conventional medicine, homoeopathic prescriptions can also usually play a part in further assisting in their therapy. In many conditions homoeopathy may well be the only medicine required, in many others it can be safely combined with appropriate non-homoeopathic medicines.

However, there are some conditions where at this stage in our knowledge, homoeopathy cannot offer an adequate medicine and conventional medical treatment will be required. A clear example is 'replacement therapy'. At present homoeopathic doctors do not have a preparation that can replace the need for such medicines as thyroxine, or insulin in patients unable to produce such substances in the natural manner. There is not a suitable homoeopathic medicine for patients regularly needing insulin injections for diabetes or thyroxine tablets for myxoedema.

There are, however, other conditions for which conventional medicine has little to offer where homoeopathy has often been found useful. Examples are chronic catarrh and sinusitis. Sometimes conventional medicine can help reduce such a problem, but not always. Many times homoeopathy has reduced these unpleasant symptoms. Often patients seek homoeopathic help when other treatment has failed to give them the relief for which they were looking. Common examples here, in addition to the arthritis and sinusitis previously mentioned, are long-lasting skin disorders such as eczema and dermatitis; bowel and bladder problems sometimes referred to as irritable bowel or bladder; hay fever, migraine and pre-menstrual tension. These are just a few examples illustrating the wide range of problems for which homoeopathic treatment is frequently sought and found useful. There are of course many others.

Psychiatric Disorders

Homoeopathic prescribers are often asked if they can help patients with psychiatric disorders. Most homoeopathic doctors advise that this form of medicine is unlikely to be of much help in such complex disorders as schizophrenia or manic-depressive illness. However, in the less dramatic but often similarly distressing difficulties that arise through recurrent experiences of depression or anxiety, homoeopathic treatment may well be a great help to the patients concerned. An appropriate homoeopathic remedy can often help a patient overcome mild or moderate degrees of such reactions and reduce or even avert their need for the stronger types of anti-depressant or anxiety relieving medicines often advised in conventional psychiatry. But here again a note of caution may be needed. If a patient has severe depressive illness, for instance, one associated with mistaken beliefs, known technically as delusions, or with strong negative thoughts and suicidal plans, they usually require more help than can be given by homoeopathic medicine. These are complex disease patterns for which various other lines of therapy may at present be more appropriate. The situation with such strong reactions and disease patterns is different from the mild or moderate depressive reactions where homoeopathy may be a very useful therapy.

A combination of therapies that has often been reported to be of particular help has been the associated use of homoeopathic treatment and psychotherapy. It is now widely acknowledged that increased understanding of how symptoms have developed, of conflicts contributing to them and of ways in which habitual anxieties can be changed, can be a very helpful therapy. Diseases likely to be helped by this approach include many with an apparent physical emphasis as well as those that clearly involve emotional stress. If we recall again that thoughts, feelings and physical processes are constantly interacting within us and contributing to our physical state it is easier to accept that an appropriate form of psychotherapeutic help can often reduce symptoms of diseases with physical as well as psychological effects. An increase of self-understanding can facilitate a redirection of body energies in a way that works towards health. Some of the techniques widely used in psychotherapy are intended to help patients release painful memories retained from past events. At times there is a need to express emotional memories not adequately released in the past.

For example, a young woman who developed severe anxiety symptoms after being shut in an underground train in a tunnel for about an hour, found out later in working on her difficulties that she had also experienced a similar severe panic on at least two previous occasions. The first one, she recalled, was a childhood experience of being shut in a cupboard. The second was her memory of being born. Releasing at least some of the fear felt in those previous experiences, but not adequately dealt with at the time, enabled her to overcome her more recent anxiety reactions. The experience in the underground train had opened up the earlier memories. In order to overcome the anxieties provoked she not only worked on them in a psychotherapeutic manner, but also had homoeopathic treatment. With the help of the combined therapies she steadily overcame the anxiety reaction. It was an example of the use of the two therapies as a complement to each another, and above all, to the motivation of the patient using their help.

Sometimes such reactions have been overcome by patients using homoeopathic help without the addition of defined psychotherapy. Others have worked through such difficulties using psychotherapy but without homoeopathy. However, in the experience of many prescribers, therapists and patients, the combined use of therapies has often been found more helpful than using either technique alone. This is not surprising. Both therapies are aiming at helping to overcome disease by assisting a re-integration of personal energy patterns. In colloquial terms both are aiming to help a person get back together on their own chosen course. Psychotherapy is aiming towards this goal through seeking a greater understanding of personal processes and therefore increased individual direction of personal responses. It is sometimes suggested that homoeopathic medicine can have a similar effect, a correct *similia* being another aid to integration of a person's various functions. One idea is that the medicine acts as a type of mirror, reminds a body of its particular state and helps re-integration. Clearly such an idea is a hypothesis and cannot be tested by ordinary objective assessments. But it is an interesting line of thought and can be pursued by logical deduction. Hence it can be argued that since both homoeopathy and psychotherapy are pursuing a similar end in a similar way they are well suited as mutually complementary.

Homoeopathy and Acupuncture

Acupuncture is another method of therapy that is sometimes said to work by assisting re-integration of hidden energy patterns as well as those more easily seen in our bodies. This therapy has similarly been found useful by many practitioners and patients, especially when combined with homoeopathy. Like many other methods of treatment acupuncture can at times be a cardinal means for treating disease. But in many other conditions its combination with homoeopathy or other appropriate therapy is even more advantageous to a patient.

The Dietary Aspect

The therapies discussed so far are methods of redirecting the energies already constituting our bodies. Another important approach concerns the input, the energy coming into them as food and drink. A car given parrafin will quickly misbehave. Similarly our bodies need the fuel appropriate to them.

In recent years there has been a lot of discussion about diets. No longer are they regarded mainly as a method of adding or reducing weight. Instead they are discussed in detail in relation to a wide range of diseases. The media frequently carry reports of various diets alleged to help conditions as various as rheumatoid arthritis, multiple sclerosis, migraine, eczema and cancer. At times this has been pursued with vigour, and many different diets have been advised in the popular press. Although some patients report benefits after following such dietary advice, others have been confused by conflicting recommendations. Often doctors are asked today 'which diet is the best one for me now?' In some diseases dietary advice is obviously important and likely to be similar from a large number of doctors. A ready example is diabetes where restriction of refined sugar is advised. But even for this disease dietary advice has been modified in recent years with less emphasis on calorie counting and more on the fibre content. Another disease where there is general agreement about diet is hypertension, or raised blood-pressure. Patients with this problem are usually advised to reduce their salt intake, and, if they are overweight, to lose weight. But with many other diseases there is generally less agreement about a diet likely to assist the therapy. For instance, for migraine, if a patient reads the popular press searching for opinions on this subject, he could at times find a different diet advised almost daily.

The wide variety of diets claimed by individuals to help

arthritis, migraine or many other diseases indicates an important principle that is also fundamental to homoeopathy; namely, the individuality of disease and therapy. Many years ago, Dr Clarke, an English homoeopathic doctor to whom there has been reference in earlier chapters, wrote 'Homoeopathy is the art of individualizing'. A basic principle of homoeopathy is the emphasis on trying to understand the needs of an individual patient as they occur now. In other words, the aim is to see him as an individual with certain symptoms, rather than defining him according to a disease label. Again this was referred to in earlier chapters, particularly when the methods of prescribing were outlined. As was said then, two children with hay fever may have apparently similar symptoms but may be reacting to them in very different ways. In homoeopathy their general reactions as well as their particular symptoms would be noted and different remedies probably advised. It emphasizes the individual nature of a disease. A similar principle applies in the selection of diets. In many diseases it is unwise to generalize. Instead there is a need for individual patients to discover which diet helps them and then use it wisely. A correct diet is an important complement to homoeopathy or any other therapy.

But whilst such individual assessment and use of diet is important, there are also some general principles that can be applied to many if not most of us. One way of thinking about diet is to remember that we eat food to obtain energy to maintain our body. For man that energy comes from food that originally comes from the sun. If the food is vegetable in nature, it is solar energy absorbed into a plant form. If it is meat it is from an animal which has eaten plants or perhaps other animals which have eaten plants. If it is a mineral ingredient of the diet, such as minute doses of various salts that are needed for healthy function of our bodies, then even these have come originally from the sun when long, long ago it was thrown off from the solar mass. At some stage in its development all our food has come from the sun. From this some people argue that plants with the solar energy and natural minerals they incorporate are less modified than if they have also been eaten and processed by animals. It is a rationale that some people use to support their preference for a vegetarian diet. But whatever diet we pursue, its energy value will be higher if the food is fresh. In addition, many dieticians argue that a diet as free as possible from chemical preservatives is better for our bodies.

In short, therefore, as a general guide, many prescribers recommend a simple fresh diet with as few chemical additives as possible. A further generalization is to advise plenty of chewing and unhurried eating. Within such generalization it is our own business to discover which food suits us best and then to use it as we will.

Whatever therapy we use, and whichever diet we take, they are always a complement to our own will and interest. As was said earlier in this chapter, if the will is set towards recovery there is more of a unified movement as body energies, and therapies used, together orientate towards health. The role of the individual will is fundamentally important. We do ourselves a great disservice if we put so much emphasis on help that appears to come from outside our body that we forget the resources that we can mobilize within it. We can co-operate with treatment, using this and an appropriate diet in an intelligent manner. We can check our own responses to treatment and discuss it with doctors or other therapists whose job it is to offer advice. If we choose to do so we can use the experience to learn more about the workings of our own bodies and how to help them keep healthy.

Disease can be an important provocation to stir us to learn more about our bodies. We can ask – what, when and why? What has happened, where is it focused, why did it occur? Such questions can help us develop a healthy interest in how our bodies are made and how they function. Of course a negative obsession with disease is not helpful. We do not want a negative preoccupation with illness. That would be like wearing very restricting blinkers, or a sort of tunnel effect. In contrast to such restriction, intelligent questioning can be a way of learning and opening up new understanding for the patient and his therapist. It can make all of us think more deeply about what is happening in health and disease. It is possible to have a healthy interest in disease.

Another useful aid to therapy is an interest in other events. Even though a patient may be lying in bed feeling ill it can be stimulating and refreshing to hear reports from visitors of their activities. Awakening a patient's interest, perhaps in a sport he has enjoyed, a place he has visited or a book he has valued, can usefully help healing from disease. An example of this has been the recently publicized use of favourite recordings to help stimulate the memory and interest of patients unconscious from road accidents. It comes back again to the idea that our bodies are energy patterns. When the flow of our thought, feeling and physical energy is directed in pursuit of something that interests us, it means there is a more convergent activity than if we are drifting without consciously applying ourselves to something. Body energy patterns need directing, then they are like water channelled and supporting life. If they are not directed, they tend to flow according to whims of the moment and are often more like an erratic flood. The interest may be in an activity, such as reading, talking with a friend, or listening to a play. Or it may be in resting and relaxing and seeing how that can help our bodies. But whatever it is, if it is pursued with interest it helps unite body energies and can usefully work together with other aids for healing.

It is often said that disease is dis-ease. That it is a disturbance of the easy interaction of a healthy body. It follows from this idea that treatment is aimed at restoring the balanced interaction; that is, to overcome the dis-ease. The use of medicine to help correct an imbalance, surgery to remove a particularly troublesome area, or acupuncture to help redirect a healthy flow, can all be enhanced by the interest of the patient in his own recovery and in events around him.

Whether we are patients or prescribers, an intelligent questioning of what is happening in disease and treatment is an important way of learning about ourselves. Some philosophers have said that the search for such knowledge is the highest aim for man. One of the early Greek philosophers put it strongly when he said, 'the unexamined life is not worth living'. A growing understanding of how our bodies work has often been assisted by an appropriate questioning of disease, why it occurs and how it can be treated. A patient who had a severe anxiety illness learnt so much through questioning what provoked her symptoms, how her body functioned and why her family reacted in particular ways, that some years later she said that she was thankful for the experience.

There is often talk of aiming for *recovery* from disease. Arguably, the greater need is to aim to use it, at least as much, for *discovery*. Even patients with diseases as serious and unpleasant as some forms of cancer have at times said they are thankful for the experience because they have learnt so much through it. This is not easy, but it finds a meaning in what otherwise is likely to be a meaningless and therefore even more difficult experience.

The questioning of disease, how it occurs and how it can be treated often leads patients having homoeopathic treatment to ask how it works. This is not easily answered. Long ago Hahnemann insisted that homoeopathy was founded on clear principles that included reference to how the medicines worked. Although Hahnemann discouraged *speculation* about how treatment might work, he applied himself very carefully in his writings to a precise *rationale* of how homoeopathic medicines help towards recovery from disease. The next chapter will refer to some of the ideas that he discussed in relation to this important question. It will also include some discussion of how they compare with some of the newer theories of healing.

Chapter 7

How Does it Work?

A question commonly asked when homoeopathy is being discussed is 'how does it work?' Sometimes it is suggested that this question is best forgotten. Some homoeopaths say that since practice shows the effectiveness of the medicines, such questions are unnecessary. This is not the attitude adopted by Hahnemann who recurrently wrote that in order to treat disease appropriately we need an understanding first of disease processes, secondly a knowledge of the medicines that can treat them and, thirdly, a knowledge of how to put these two together. That principle is as valid today as it was for Hahnemann. His insistence that homoeopathy is a 'rational' system of medicine, as well as his copious writings on the subject, imply that for him it was founded on principles deduced before they are tested and verified in the sickroom. For him, the consideration of 'how does homoeopathy work?' was clearly of fundamental importance.

These principles are still valid today. Human beings have a particular capacity for reason and understanding. Since health implies wholeness, it follows therefore that complete health implies appropriate use of our capacity for understanding the events that concern us, and that includes those constituting our own bodies. In relation to health and disease it implies the need appropriately to question what causes them, rather than merely passively swallowing pills in the hope that they will correct a problem. Examining the question, 'how does homoeopathy work?' can be a particularly useful way of learning not only about this form of medical practice, but about how a human body functions in every moment. Such understanding can then increase personal chances of staying healthy. Someone who understands the working of cars is more likely to be able to correct their faults than a person who knows next to nothing about them. Similarly, with our bodies. The more we understand them, the quicker we can make appropriate adjustments to help them remain healthy.

Let us look first at Hahnemann's theory about how homoeopathy works and then secondly consider some more recent ideas and discoveries that relate to it.

The 'Vital Force'

The theory developed by Hahnemann included reference to the 'vital force'. In his day the idea was widely held that an invisible energy operated in all beings and governed their visible forms and activities. It was thought of as an unseen component of every organism, operating in all beings, yet unique in each one. It was a way of expressing an understanding that the activity seen with the ordinary eyes was only a part of man and that this outwardly visible structure was directed all the time by an inward invisible force. In his attempt to understand disease Hahnemann deduced that symptoms reported by patients were produced by disturbances in this unseen vital force. He expressed this opinion many times. Examples of it are found for instance in paragraphs 11 and 12 of the sixth edition of the *Organon* where he firmly states his opinion that the symptoms of which patients complain are the visible effects produced by unseen changes in the vital force.

Hahnemann was writing before the discovery of bacteria and viruses. In his day such agents were unknown and disease was generally thought to be transmitted by a non-material influence for which the term 'miasm' was sometimes used, and which he suggested disrupted the vital force. Today there is no exact translation for the word 'miasm'. The idea it represents has unfortunately been largely displaced by the demonstration of the existence of disease-provoking agents such as bacteria and viruses. This demonstration has tended to reinforce an erroneous entity concept of disease and the term 'miasm' has largely been unnecessarily dropped from our vocabulary. However, it is also widely acknowledged that factors as subtle as hereditary traits or psychological processes can also influence vulnerability to disease. Arguably this is the miasm theory re-worded.

Haemophilia is a well-known example of a distinct hereditary disease. Other diseases such as some thyroid disorders tend to show a familiar pattern. Depression is a well-known psychological process often associated with various physical symptoms. It is arguable that such descriptions imply processes akin to the miasm theory widely held in Hahnemann's day and frequently employed by him when discussing the causes of disease. He emphasized the role of such forces transmitted by one individual to another in provoking disturbances of the individual vital force and therefore resulting in the symptoms of disease. A long footnote to paragraph 11 of the *Organon* is one example of Hahnamann's interpretation of this theory.

But, at the same time, Hahnemann was also working towards ideas that came very close to the viral or bacterial theory of disease causation to be evolved later in history. His writings of the causes of cholera include a comparison of the cholera miasm to a 'murderous organism attached to man's skin, hair or clothing . . . and transferred invisibly from man to man'. He anticipates the discovery of the vibrio later found to be transmitted by contaminated water in outbreaks of cholera. But although his writings may be said to anticipate the bacterial theory of disease development, they still strongly express his opinion that even such agents would produce their effects through a dynamic effect on the vital force. Once disrupted it is this unseen aspect of the human body that Hahnemann says produces the visible changes recognized as indications of disease.

The next stage in Hahnemann's argument is to say that as the cause of disease is such a dynamic or immaterial force, a similarly dynamic and non-material agent will be required to correct it. The 'likes for likes' theory, as the *similia* principle is sometimes described, implies not only that the symptoms of a disease are similar to those the appropriate medicine can produce, but also that the medicine required is of a similar quality to the disturbance producing a disease. Such a dynamic medicine, he argues, is prepared or unveiled by potentization; that is, the serial dilution and vigorous shaking developed by him and still used today in the preparation of homoeopathic medicines. Such a dynamic radical, he argued, was then capable of interacting with the disturbed vital force to help restore health.

He then suggests how this correction was produced. Again his discussion focused on the activity of the vital force which he said could produce disease if disturbed, or maintain health when its own function was correct. He argued that when disease occurred the vital force opposed the disturbance within itself in an attempt to overcome it. But if the symptoms did not clear, this meant that the resistance to it had been inadequate or inappropriate in some way. The aim of therapy was therefore appropriately to assist this reaction. He called it a 'counter-revolution' and said it helped to restore the correct state of the vital force and therefore of the physical organs which it directs. In other words the aim of therapy was to stimulate the opposition against disease by assisting the vital force to counter its own disruption and therefore restore a healthy balance.

That is a basic outline of the theory. Now for more detail.

Hahnemann's writings include careful discussions of why a

homoeopathic medicine – that is, one prescribed according to the law of similars – was best suited to provoke the required reaction from the vital force.

His argument was that because the medicine could provoke a similar symptom picture to that occurring in a disease, it was also capable of stimulating an appropriate reaction from the vital force. In other words, when a correct homoeopathic medicine is taken by a patient, it disturbs the vital force in a manner similar to that occurring in the disease and at the same time provokes a further reaction from it. He reasoned that the potentized medicine presented a stimulus to the vital force, not only similar to that occurring in the natural disease process, but also stronger because of the potentization. This in turn, he said, heightened the counter-revolution from the vital force. This heightened reaction against the medicinal stimulus then also worked against the disease similar to it. This increased reaction could then overcome the original disease. He also argued that because the medicine had been potentized it produced a reaction that was shorter as well as stronger than that of the disease, and that this also aided a prompt return to health.

It is an interesting theory which can be compared to some of the ideas discussed currently in an attempt to explain how healing of disease occurs. There is a lot of talk to-day about antibodies to diseases. The media and popular press frequently carry reports of how antibodies play a part in overcoming disease and restoring healthy function. Such antibodies are protein products of cells contributing to immune responses. They are said to oppose the agents causing diseases and therefore to check their development. They could be likened to an army roused to combat an invader. In some diseases measurements are made of these immune proteins and recorded as 'antibody titres'. A rising titre can be a sign of active infection. It is a way of assessing the organic response to a disease process.

Hahnemann's theory of opposition from the vital force can

be compared with such an insight. Laboratory studies demonstrate that in certain diseases there is organic opposition to the intruding infection. It is arguable that this is one particular gross example of the bodies own opposition to disease, comparable to and determined by the counter-revolution of the vital force. It is paradoxical that Hahnamann advised prescribing a medicine capable of producing a *similia* effect in order to provoke a suitable and stronger *opposing* reaction. The aim of the similimum was to produce a counter-revolution of the vital force. One indication of that opposing reaction occuring may well be the antibodies, the level of which can be measured today in certain diseases.

'Inner Recognition'

Another way of comparing Hahnemann's theories of healing with those of modern medicine is to use a psychological model. In pyschotherapy, techniques are at times employed that are intended to assist a personal recognition of a patient's own previously unacknowledged responses. This can be an aim in group or individual psychotherapy with the therapist or members of a group feeding back to a person the impression they give. For instance, a therapist or another group member may sometimes comment after someone has spoken of an experience, 'to me you sound angry about that', or sad, or happy, whatever the reaction might appear to be. It is often only when such impressions are discussed that the person recounting the experience gains more insight into how he himself is actually feeling about it. It is all too easy not to notice how we feel about things that happen to us. Often people will say, 'I don't feel angry about it' when they are tight lipped and clenching their fingers as they say it.

Feedback can often help recognition. Only after recognition of a reaction can there be a deliberate attempt to understand it and perhaps consciously to change it. Such feedback often occurs in ordinary conversation with family and friends. A simple example is a mother making her own expression look fed up and cross when she wants to show a disconsolate child how they appear. It occurs, too, in conversation when someone says, for instance, 'you are so down-hearted that I am feeling it'. Such feedback does not always need the refined techniques of group or individual therapy, although these can be an important additional aid to clarifying the less obvious reactions.

This sort of feedback, whatever the environment in which it is offered, can help a person recognize their own behaviour traits. Only when such traits are acknowledged can the person showing them consciously choose either to continue or to change them. The recognition is essential prior to the further step of deliberately continuing or modifying a behaviour pattern and therefore of realizing greater self-understanding.

The effect of a correct homoeopathic medicine can be likened to this process. It is as if the medicinal stimulus acts as a further reminder to the person of the disease process and its behavioural effects, and by heightening the picture helps an inner recognition that assists the personal response to it. In other words, a disease process is heightened to provoke recognition of its effects and appropriate reaction against it. A further stage in the argument deduces that taking personal charge of reactions in this way implies increased co-ordination of our energies and therefore another step towards healthy balance. It is like an army organizing itself for a battle.

Initiatory Forces

The successive editions of the *Organon* show how Hahnemann continually developed his ideas about the essential determinants of health, disease and therapy. The fifth and sixth editions contain frequent references, not only to the effects of the vital force in producing health or disease, but of even more subtle factors such as 'spirit-like essences' or perhaps better translated today, initiatory forces. He argued that these 'spirit-like' forms were the inner determinants of medicines and that they were released or unveiled through potentization.

Like many researchers before him Hahnemann was trying to understand the essential causes of events. He appears to work through to the idea that these are spirit-like forms, the highest determinants of a heirarchy of causes seen in human activity. He suggests that initiatory forces, or, as they are sometimes translated, conceptual essences, come first, that the higher reason is developed in man as a capacity to understand such determinant forces, and that the gross physical processes are their embodiment. These are not easy concepts to discuss. Perhaps it is partly because of this that they are often excluded from discussions of homoeopathy. But if we are attempting to understand how this method of treatment works it is important to include reference to them.

It appears that Hahnemann's understanding was that these initiatory spirit-like essences are the primary determinants of existence. That is, that they set in motion a process which, although it may be modified by other stimuli later, actually begins with them. These unseen forms, he deduces, originally determine the gross, ordinarily seen forms of animals, vegetables or minerals. In the course of its existence the gross visible expression of the unseen form may be modified by other stimuli, although its prime mover remains the spirit-like essence. An obvious example of such modification is when physical violence breaks the product.

When Hahnemann applies such theories to human health and disease he suggests that a subtle form is again the original determinant of an individual person's configuration, that this governs the physical growth, but that its presentation may be modified by a wrong diet, poor sanitation or other causes of disease which may include other initiatory force forms unassimilable to the individual. One way of illustrating this theory is to compare it to the pattern in an acorn that determines that, given appropriate nourishment, it will become an oak tree. The structure of the tree and the phases through which it passes are expansions of that original pattern. The healthy life cycle reveals the pattern. However, its expression may be modified if the growing form does not receive sufficient light or water, or is affected by disease or physical violence. Although such factors may affect its gross appearance, the original determinant is the primary pattern, or using Hahnemann's terms, the spirit-like essence. Without this the process would not start.

Such spiritual essences, Hahnemann argues, are the original determinants, or prime movers, of human existence, as well as of other forms. He deduces that they can be recognized by the higher mind or reason of man who is also given sufficient intelligence to understand and employ them in assisting healing.

In applying such insights therapeutically he suggests that the stimulus from a rightly prescribed potentized medicine is a way of applying a conceptual essence. As noted earlier, he deduced that potentization revealed the essential form of a medicine. Hahnemann suggests that in an appropriate situation, this essential form presented in the medicine can provoke the vital force in a way that will help restore physical and psychological health.

Such ideas refer back again to Hahnemann's three-part assessment of the knowledge needed for adequate therapy. As he said many times, therapy requires first a knowledge of disease, then of the powers hidden within medicines and, thirdly, of how to apply these judiciously to assist healing. His understanding that disease is caused by subtle forces implies that a similar agent is required to correct it. It is to be similar in kind as well as in the effects it is able to produce in healthy volunteers. Such ideas clearly occupied Hahnemann for a lifetime. They have also continued to provoke many thinkers who have followed him and have attempted to pursue and further develop the understanding he was seeking to convey in his writings.

As was noted in an earlier chapter, the understanding of any subject needs to be progressive. The alternative is a stagnant repetition of increasingly out-dated concepts. It is vital for the continuance of homoeopathy that we attempt to follow Hahnemann's example and persevere in asking what are the causes of disease, the determinants of the effects of medicines and how these insights can be applied in therapy.

The final chapter will include reference to some of the ways in which such questions are being pursued today.

Chapter 8

Reflections on Homoeopathy

It is often said of medicine today that the research that appears to clarify an understanding of some of its concerns, produces at least as many questions as it answers. People involved with other studies will say the same thing about their particular interests. In subjects as diverse as cookery, computing and conjuring, as well as in medicine, the more we learn, the more we realize there is to learn.

Homoeopathy is another particularly clear example of this principle. We may start off by discovering that it is a form of medical practice, that its name implies the *similia* principle fundamental to it, and that in prescribing such medicines very small doses are generally employed. We may then go on to learn that in order to find out which homoeopathic medicine may be required for a patient, a prescriber is likely to ask many and varied questions, not only about the particular symptoms that the patient expects to report, but about his past history, his likes and dislikes now, his general body responses and even sometimes about his hopes for the future. We will discover that homoeopathic prescribing is orientated towards a wide review of the condition of a patient requesting treatment and that a medicine selected is frequently chosen at least as much for the patient generally as for the particular symptoms he presents. All of this can be very interesting, and at each stage in the discovery, if we allow it to happen, more and more questions come to mind.

There are many aspects to this study that warrant increasing research. Three particular areas often questioned are the details of how the medicines are produced, how the needs of a particular patient are assessed and a medicine selected for him, and why or how it achieves its effect. Such questions were asked by Hahnemann and are still being pursued today. They have far-reaching implications, not only concerning the practice of homoeopathy as a method of treating disease, but for our progressive understanding of the determinants of life and health, disease and death.

One of the particularly challenging aspects of homoeopathic medicine concerns the effectiveness of the miniscule doses it frequently employs. This aspect of the practice appears to contradict the general trend of prescribing in other forms of conventional medical practice. In many conditions patients know that with orthodox prescriptions if one tablet is not sufficient to give the required help, an increased dose may be advised. Toothache is an example. Most people treating this may try one pain-relieving tablet and if this does not help they double the dose. For many conditions, if the initial prescription proves insufficient, the patient may well be advised to take twice as much.

Homoeopathic prescribing is very different from this. Here, if a prescription appears not to help, and a prescriber checks it and still believes it is an appropriate *similia* for the patient, he may well advise a dosage that is much reduced from the original. That reduction may be as much as a million times less in terms of gross assessments (if they are valid here). For instance, an adult with influenza whose symptoms have not improved after taking *Aconite 6c* may be advised to take a *30c* preparation. In this situation the extra degree of dilution is far greater than a mere millionth. It illustrates the paradox of homoeopathy. At times progressively finer stimuli are applied in order to treat gross effects of disease. Instead of doubling doses, homoeopathic prescribers often minimize them.

Subtle Influences

If we allow our questioning minds to run on from this observation we can enter some very interesting and thought provoking areas. Western society places an emphasis on material assessments and aims. Our bodies are generally understood, or at least attempted to be so, in terms of gross organs, with defined cells, which in turn are made up of defined gross elements, all functioning together to make a healthy unit, we hope. Sometimes allowance is made for the influence of thoughts, feelings or other aspects of the 'psyche'. But even so the emphasis in contemporary Western medicine is generally on the seen rather than the unseen. One of the challenges of homoeopathy is that it provokes re-examination of this emphasis. Homoeopathy shows that prescriptions containing doses of medicine so small that they elude even high-powered microscopes or other laboratory methods of detection, produce a distinct biological effect. This observation can usefully provoke the question, 'how do they do it?' Here is an example of stimuli too small for detection by ordinary laboratory techniques, yet sufficient to help change the course of diseases in children, adults and animals. It challenges researchers to look again at previous assessments of the determinants of health and to allow for the effects of forces too elusive for gross assessment.

Such researches relate closely to ideas often presented in psychology and psychiatry. It is widely acknowledged today that thoughts and feelings can change gross physical activity. Ordinary people know that good news or bad can strongly influence the way they feel and how they function physically. This is a simple observation, but one that has far-reaching implications. One of the implications is that in every moment, not just in times of crisis, the thoughts and feelings allowed to operate within people actually contribute to their physical health or disease. Obviously there is more to disease than thinking about it, but in allowing for the effects of other factors there is also the need not to forget the influence of thought and feeling. In every moment such subtle influences can help or hinder the physical activities of our bodies.

Perhaps Hahnemann had such thoughts in mind when he referred to homoeopathic medicines in their ultradilute and succussed form as, using the German words 'geistartigen Wesen', now sometimes translated as 'conceptual essence'. The term concept is often used for a thought form. Perhaps Hahnemann had in mind a comparison between the effects of thoughts in determining gross physical activity, and the capacity for the very fine stimulus of the medicine to effect a physical change. His writings in the *Organon* appear to imply this.

Both in the time of Hahnemann and today, homoeopathy has challenged materialistically biased assessments of disease and therapy. It provokes researchers to look behind the façade of gross anatomy, physiology and pathology in hopes of learning something more about the subtle forces that direct them. Of course, the assessment of gross changes is important. Greater understanding of organic, cellular and chemical changes is obviously important and helpful. But so too is a progressive questioning and understanding of the influences that direct such superficial levels of function. As many writers in all ages have reminded us, we need to look through or beyond the ordinarily seen processes in hopes of trying to understand their causes.

Understanding the Determinants of Disease and Therapy

The search for insight into causes was another theme recurrently pursued by Hahnemann, and again is similarly important today. Understanding of the causes of disease is a prerequisite for its adequate treatment. The six editions of the *Organon* testify to ways in which throughout his long life Hahnemann continued searching for an understanding of the causes of disease. They show his progressive clarification of an idea that the patterns of forces that he called spirit-like or conceptual essences determine the gross appearance of plants, animal and mineral products from which medicines can be obtained. These patterns, he suggested were released or unveiled through potentization and presented in a form that could stimulate the similarly subtle energies of the human body and help provoke healing. His search for causes led him to the realms of philosophy and wide-ranging yet detailed ideas about the subtle as well as gross determinants of life and health. His awareness of the importance of recognizing all aspects in the heirarchy of causes of disease is shown by his frequent references to the need for correct diet and hygiene as well as to reflections on spirit-like essences.

The attempts to understand more about the heirarchy of causes of disease and its treatment is illustrated today by the various types of research being pursued in hopes of discovering more about homoeopathy. Some of the research projects include studies of the effects of homoeopathic medicines in particular diseases. Earlier chapters contained references to two such studies, one done in Glasgow assessing homoeopathic treatment in patients with rheumatoid arthritis and another from the Royal London Homoeopathic Hospital assessing the response of children treated for recurrent ear, nose and throat infections. Many other studies of this nature are still going on to-day.

Another type of research being pursued in the Royal London Homoeopathic Hospital research unit concerns the effects of potentized medicines on wheat seedlings and yeast cells. Clearly this is a different form of research from clinical studies with patients, but it is usefully illustrating the effects on cell growth on the minute doses of stimulus in potentized medicine. In other centres research is being carried out concerning the detailed physio-chemical properties of such highly dilute preparations as are often used in homoeopathic medicine. A detailed review of current research procedures relevant to homoeopathy is beyond the scope of this book. These few examples are given merely as an introduction to this important aspect of the subject. They are mentioned merely to illustrate the many lines of research that are relevant to a progressive understanding of homoeopathy, the nature of its medicines and how a *similia* prescribed in a minute dosage can be an effective agent in arousing the forces that can be consciously employed to help correct a disease.

At times homoeopathy has been described as old-fashioned and harmlessly ineffective. Many patients and prescribers refute this. They have found it highly effective and, as valid today as it was two hundred years ago. Homoeopathy is not an out-dated relic of pre-scientific medicine. It is an effective therapy with an important contribution to make to modern medicine. It can help allay the unpleasant symptoms of many diseases. At the same time it can usefully provoke important questions concerning a far reaching and fundamental study of the determinants of health and disease and how such dilute preparations widely used in homoeopathy can achieve therapeutic effects. Arguably homoeopathy can be a vital complement to conventional medical practice. Hopefully, as time goes on, insight into the unseen factors that govern our health and disease will increase. It is also to be hoped that with the greater understanding there will be more respect for the therapeutics founded on the operation of such subtle determinants of gross organic effects.

Many years ago Hahnemann introduced the term 'potentization' to describe the process by which homoeopathic medicines were, and still are, prepared. It was deliberately intended to remind its users that the processes of serial dilution and succussion revealed previously hidden essential powers in the sources of the medicines. The term 'potency' was similarly intended to emphasize the subtle powers presented in such medicines. Hopefully, today we are moving towards a greater recognition of the important implications of these terms.

Useful Addresses

Main Homoeopathic Associations

National Center for Homoeopathy
1500 Massachusettes Avenue, N.W.
Suite 41
Washington D.C. 20005
(Tel: 202–223–6182)
Publishes a directory of licensed health professionals in the
U.S. and Canada who practice homeopathic medicine.

International Foundation for Homeopathy
1141 Northwest Market Street
Seattle, WA 98107
(Tel: 206–789–7327)

United States Homeopathic Association
6560 Backlick Road
Springfield, VA 22150
(Tel: 703–569–5311)

American Association of Homeopathic Pharmacists
Willard Eldredge, President
P.O. Box 2273
Falls Church, VA 22042
(Tel: 717–685–7085)

A wide range of books on homeopathic medicine is available from:

Thorsons Publishers Inc.
377 Park Avenue South
New York, NY 10016

Index